Testicular Tumors
Management and Treatment

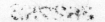

Testicular Tumors
Management and Treatment

Edited by

Lawrence H. Einhorn, M.D.

School of Medicine
Indiana University
Indianapolis, Indiana

MASSON Publishing USA, Inc.

New York • Paris • Barcelona • Milan • Mexico City • Rio de Janeiro

ISBN 0-89352-078-0

Library of Congress Catalog Card Number: 79-89999

Printed in the United States of America

CANCER MANAGEMENT

Luther W. Brady and Vincent T. DeVita, Jr., Series Editors

PINEAL TUMORS
Edited by Henry H. Schmidek (1977)

THE CHEMISTRY OF
RADIOPHARMACEUTICALS
Edited by Ned D. Heindel, H. Donald Burns, Takashi Honda
and Luther W. Brady (1978)

TESTICULAR TUMORS:
MANAGEMENT AND TREATMENT
Edited by Lawrence H. Einhorn (1980)

CLINICAL ONCOLOGY:
THE FOUNDATIONS OF
CURRENT PATIENT MANAGEMENT
(AND SELECTED THERAPEUTIC
DEVELOPMENTS)
Edited by Jesús Vicente, Hernán Cortes-Funes,
Pablo Viladiu, and Franco M. Muggia (1980)

INTRODUCTION

ALTHOUGH testicular cancer is a relatively rare disease (only 2,500–3,000 expected cases in 1979), it is an extremely important malignancy for many reasons. First of all, it is the commonest carcinoma in men 15 to 35 years of age, and thus, it is an extremely important disease because of the potential loss of productive years of life. Secondly, it is one of the few tumors where the clinician has the luxury of serum markers (serum beta subunit human chorionic gonadotropin and alphafetoprotein) to help direct initial and future therapy and to help determine completeness of tumor eradication. Dr. Lange's chapter (Chap. 4) clearly brings into sharp focus past, present, and future directions involving HCG and alphafetoprotein, and will prove to be informative and illuminating to all readers. Thirdly, there has been worldwide controversy as to the preferrable method of therapy for clinical Stage I or II nonseminomatous testicular cancer. In the United States, "standard" therapy has been orchiectomy followed by retroperitoneal lymphadenectomy, a procedure that usually causes sterility because of interruption of the sympathetic plexus and concomitant failure of ejaculation. In Europe, orchiectomy followed by definitive radiotherapy is the preferred method of treatment. Although sterility is uncommon compared to lymphadenectomy, such irradiation may have considerably more serious consequences. Since a finite proportion of clinical Stage I and II patients with nonseminomatous testicular cancer are destined to relapse, and thus require chemotherapy, it is crucially important that initial therapy be employed in such a matter so as not to compromise future potentially curative chemotherapy. Unfortunately, patients with prior radiotherapy clearly have a decreased tolerance for aggressive chemotherapy, a factor which well might compromise future survival should relapse occur. However, there is more to this argument than whether or not radiotherapy alone, surgery alone, or a combination of the two disciplines should be employed in the management of Stage I or II nonseminomatous testicular cancer. Fifty to sixty percent of patients with clinical Stage I or II disease have *pathological* Stage I disease (negative nodes following thorough bilateral retroperitoneal lymphadenectomy). Clearly such patients do not require radiotherapy *or* lymphadenectomy, as 90% of such patients were cured by radical orchiectomy alone. In the past, urologists and radiotherapists had trepidation about leaving the retroperitoneal nodes untreated in patients with clinical Stage I disease, because they knew 10–25% of such patients in reality would harbor microscopic or macroscopic disease in these nodes. However, that fear is no longer justified, as even if we do "miss" some patients with true pathological Stage II disease, the potential cure rate with chemotherapy (or surgery) should be close to 100%.

Thus, I feel we are ready for a major departure in this country in our management of clinical Stage I–II nonseminomatous tumors. Those patients who are clinical Stage I disease (normal HCG, alphafetoprotein, abdominal ultrasound, computed tomography, and/or lymphangiogram) should be subjected to a staging laparotomy only, and if the sentinel nodes and representative inspected nodes are grossly and microscopically normal, then no further therapy should be required. Such patients would not have sterility as a consequence of this procedure, and close postoperative follow-up should ensure cure rates in such patients above 95%. Obviously, the only patient who truly has a therapeutic need for lymphadenectomy and/or irradiation is the patient with Stage II disease. By following this simple guideline, we can immediately eliminate 50% of the "unnecessary" lymphadenectomies (i.e., patients with pathological Stage I).

Dr. Shipley's excellent chapter (Chap. 3) on radiotherapy is among the best and most comprehensive treatise ever published on this subject. He raises logical and excellent points in defense of irradiation instead of lymphadenectomy. Although I do not personally concur with all of his conclusions, his logic and interpretation of present data are unimpeachable. I do feel this chapter is "must reading" for urologists and chemotherapists who defend alternative approaches with equal logic and rationale. Dr. Shipley makes the statement in a less controversial area, the management of clinical Stage I and II seminoma, that "the three year disease-free survival results of radiation therapy following radical orchiectomy in patients with Stage I or II testicular seminoma are 97% and 85%, respectively, in the 767 patients reviewed and that this extraordinarily high success rate makes seminoma to date surpassed only by skin cancers as the most successfully managed group of tumors in all oncologic clinical practice." Although these results are clearly laudable, there is reason to believe that even better results can now be achieved in Stage I and II nonseminomatous tumors, and it may well be that seminoma will no longer be the most favorable germinal neoplasm, stage for stage. Primary modality therapy (orchiectomy plus retroperitoneal lymphadenectomy) can never be expected to produce the excellent results in Stage II nonseminomatous disease that can be achieved in Stage II seminoma. However, the ultimate *cure rate* may well be higher in nonseminomatous disease because of the high success rate of chemotherapy. At Indiana University, 111 of 112 patients (99.1%) with Stage I and II nonseminomatous tumors followed by our medical oncology section are currently alive and disease-free. Most of these patients were treated surgically by our urologist, Dr. John Donohue, with orchiectomy and retroperitoneal lymphadenectomy. However, some of these operations were performed outside our medical center, explaining the slight discrepancy in these figures with the data provided by Dr. Donohue's chapter (Chap. 2) on surgery. No patient had radiotherapy, and adjuvant chemotherapy was essentially not employed, although many earlier patients received postoperative actinomycin-D without any apparent benefit in the postoperative relapse rate. Although the follow-up is not "complete" in all of these patients, there is every reason to believe that a 95–99% cure rate will be accomplished in this series of patients.

Successful chemotherapy of disseminated testicular cancer has been a significant advance in medical oncology, and this subject is thoroughly covered in the appropriate chapter. Furthermore, the rationale for much of the approaches in the preceding paragraphs is based on this highly effective chemotherapy for metastatic disease. Data from Indiana University clearly support the concept that a high cure rate in disseminated testicular cancer can be attained, and it is reasonable to hypothesize that the cure rate for disseminated testicular cancer is presently 60–70%. Although other institutions have used major and minor variations in the philosophy of their chemotherapy programs, it is important to be aware of the Indiana data. Although comparison of patient populations at separate institutions is difficult, it is worth noting that the VAB regimens pioneered at Memorial Hospital or the velban-bleomycin programs from M. D. Anderson Hospital have not approached the potential cure rate with platinum + vinblastine + bleomycin.

Finally, testicular cancer stands as a "landmark tumor" in adult oncology because it is the first solid tumor to enjoy a high cure rate. This success rate is based on an apparently synergistic two drug regimen (vinblastine + bleomycin), combined with a new and unique agent, *cis*-diamminodichloroplatinum. I feel that there is optimism that future years will produce success rates in other solid tumors with continued clinical research into new combinations and active phase I and phase II agents.

CONTRIBUTORS

Bryan Burney, M.D. *Radiology, University Hospital–Indiana University Medical Center, Indianapolis, Indiana.*

John Donohue, M.D. *Urology Department, Indiana University Medical Center, Indianapolis, Indiana.*

Lawrence H. Einhorn, M.D. *Indiana University Medical Center, Indianapolis, Indiana.*

Paul Lange, M.D. *Urology Department, University of Minnesota, Minneapolis, Minnesota.*

Lawrence Roth, M.D. *Indiana University Medical Center; Pathology, University Hospital, Indianapolis, Indiana.*

William Shipley, M.D. *Radiation-Oncology, General Hospital, Boston, Massachusetts.*

Stephen D. Williams, M.D. *Indiana University Medical Center, Indianapolis, Indiana.*

CONTENTS

1

Pathology and Ultrastructure of Germinal Neoplasms of the Testis

Lawrence M. Roth, M.D.

Department of Pathology, Indiana University School of Medicine, Indianapolis, Indiana

John J. Gillespie, M.D.*

Department of Pathology, Indiana University School of Medicine, Indianapolis, Indiana

Classification and Nomenclature

PRIMARY TESTICULAR NEOPLASMS fall into two major groups: those arising from germ cells, constituting over 94% of cases; and those apparently arising from nongerminal elements, which make up the remainder.[1] The latter will not be discussed in this review except where they enter into the differential diagnosis. Germ cell tumors have been further subdivided in varied ways. One of the most popular classifications, proposed in the 1940's by Friedman and Moore[2] was based upon a study of 1000 testicular neoplasms collected at the Army Medical Museum during World War II. Each of the categories proposed represents a distinct histologic type (see Table I). This classification is relatively simple and is still widely used by clinicians. A more detailed classification was presented in the Armed Forces Institute of Pathology fascicle, *Tumors of the Male Genital Tract*, 2nd

---

* Present address: Department of Pathology, E. W. Sparrow Hospital, Lansing, Michigan.

1

Table I. Pathologic Classification of Testicular Germinal Tumors (Friedman and Moore)

1. Seminoma (analogous to the dysgerminoma of the ovary)
2. Embryonal carcinoma
3. Choriocarcinoma (similar to the uterine tumor)
4. Teratoma (analogous to ovarian dermoid)
5. Teratocarcinoma (embryonal carcinoma and teratoma)

Series[1] and in the World Health Organization International Classification of Tumours Monograph, *Histological Typing of Testicular Tumours*.[3]

The above classifications are based on the theory that both seminoma and nonseminomatous tumors originate from germ cells, and are sometimes referred to as the American Classification. Willis,[4] on the other hand, considered seminomas to be of germ cell origin and nonseminomatous tumors to be teratomas, but stated that monocellular testicular teratoma could best be designated as embryonal carcinoma. Collins and Pugh[5] and their associates in 1964 amplified Willis's classification of teratoma. The former classification is commonly referred to as the British Classification.

Teilum[6,7] has studied gonadal neoplasms for over 30 years and has been a proponent of the analogy between testicular and ovarian tumors.

In our opinion, Teilum's concepts provide the best insight into the histogenesis and interrelationship of tumors of germ cell origin (Table II). He regards seminoma as a tumor of unipotential germ cells, and embryonal carcinoma as a tumor composed of undifferentiated multipotential embryonal cells that can differ-

Table II. Histogenesis and Interrelationship of Testicular Germinal Neoplasms (Teilum)

Table III. Current Pathologic Classification of Germinal Tumors of the Testis

Germ Cell Tumors

Tumors of one histologic type
    Seminoma (Germinoma)
        Typical seminoma
        Anaplastic seminoma
        Spermatocytic seminoma
    Embryonal carcinoma
    Polyembryoma
    Yolk sac carcinoma (endodermal sinus tumor)
    Choriocarcinoma
    Teratoma
        Mature
        Immature
        With malignant transformation
        Lesions interpreted as monodermal development within a teratoma (specify)

Tumors of more than one histologic type
    Embryonal carcinoma and teratoma (teratocarcinoma)
    Other combinations (specify)

Mixed Germ Cell and Sex Cord-Stromal Tumors
    Gonadoblastoma

entiate toward either extra-embryonic or embryonic structures. His concepts seem to be more in keeping with the American Classification than the British concepts.

In this article we will use the American Classification of germ cell tumors. Our own classification is an amalgamation of the more recent classifications by American authors,[1] the work of Teilum,[7] and the World Health Organization.[3]

The soundness and practicality of this classification have been supported by an experience with over 6000 testicular tumors filed in the American Testicular Tumor Registry at the Armed Forces Institute of Pathology.[1] Two points deserve emphasis, however. Although in 60% of the cases the lesion exhibits a consistent pattern throughout, in 40% more than one pattern is encountered.[1] Dixon and Moore,[8] indeed, noted as many at 15 combinations. Moreover, although metastases also may present in pure form histologically, combinations are frequently observed. On occasion, the metastases may show a pattern not found in the primary tumor. As a second point of interest, it is noteworthy that almost 90% of the deaths resulting from metastasis occurred within two years of orchiectomy.[9] It is uncommon for a tumor-related death to occur after this period and exceedingly rare after 5 years.[9]

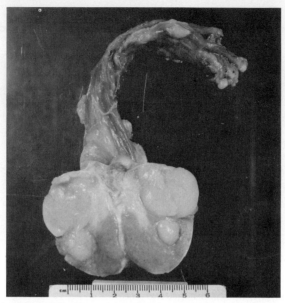

FIGURE 1.   Cut surface of the testis removed from a 62-year-old man shows partial replacement by a multinodular well-demarcated tumor with a pale uniform smooth homogeneous appearance, characteristic of seminoma.

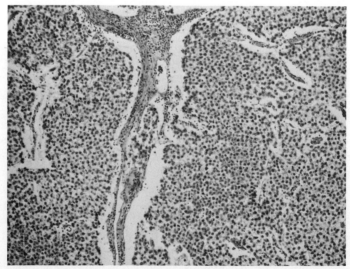

FIGURE 2.   Photomicrograph of a classical seminoma shows uniform individual germinal cells resembling spermatogonia separated by fibrous connective tissue septa infiltrated by lymphocytes. (Hematoxylin and eosin; reduced from ×100).

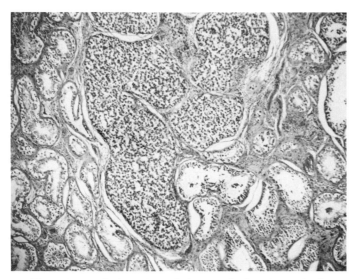

FIGURE 3.   Photomicrograph shows intratubular growth of seminoma in the same tumor depicted in Figure 2. The tubules in the center are distended with typical seminoma cells. Maturation of the cells in the innerportions of the tubules is not seen, in contrast to the appearance of normal spermatogenesis. Compressed atrophic seminiferous tubules are noted at the periphery of the tumor. (Hematoxylin and eosin; reduced from ×63).

Pathology

Seminoma (Germinoma)

Seminoma is the most frequent testicular neoplasm appearing in pure form in about 40 percent of cases.[9] It is a tumor of primitive germ cells that typically are fairly uniform and have clear cytoplasm and well-defined cell borders.[8] The identical tumor occurring in the ovary is usually referred to as dysgerminoma. The more general term, "germinoma," may be applied to these tumors occurring in either gonad or in such extragonadal sites as the retroperitoneum, mediastinum, pituitary, or pineal region. Seminomas may be further subclassified into three categories: the typical or classic form, which is by far the most common; an anaplastic variety, that accounts for fewer than 10% of cases; and a spermatocytic variety, the least common.[9] Seminoma arises more commonly than teratoid tumors in undescended testes, and tends to occur in individuals approximately 10 years older.[9] The testis may be enlarged up to 10 times its normal size, and yet its normal gonadal configuration is maintained. On section, the tumor is usually solitary and distinct from the surrounding parenchyma (Fig. 1). Its white-pink coloration contrasts with the tan-brown normal parenchyma. Although occasional small foci of necrosis appear, the surface is usually smooth and homogeneous. The occurrence of hemorrhage or cyst formation should lead one to suspect another type of neoplasm, with the exception that spermatocytic seminomas may

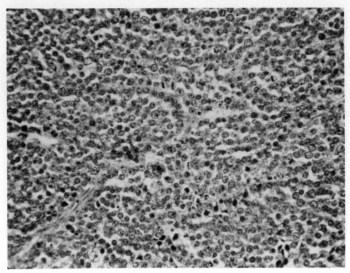

FIGURE 4.   Photomicrograph of an anaplastic seminoma shows a tumor composed of more irregular appearing germinal cells than seen in classical seminoma and at least three mitotic figures. (Hematoxylin and eosin; reduced from ×250).

contain cystic spaces. Histologically, the typical seminoma is characterized by large, uniform, round, or polyhedral cells resembling spermatogonia separated into lobules or cords by delicate fibrous tissue septa containing variable numbers of mature lymphocytes and small blood vessels (Fig. 2). The cells are not cohesive. The cytoplasm has a watery or cloudy appearance due to the presence of glycogen, but may be rather inconspicuous. Nuclei are round and moderately large, containing clumped chromatin and one or two nucleoli. Mitoses are not numerous except in the anaplastic variety. The lymphocytic component may be so dense as to obscure much of the histologic detail; in rare instances the inflammatory reaction may be granulomatous in character and simulate granulomatous orchitis, from which seminoma must be distinguished. A varied degree of fibrosis may be manifest, and this too occasionally may obscure the nature of the neoplasm. Usually the seminoma is circumscribed and set off from the normal surrounding parenchyma. On occasion, however, the parenchyma is invaded and even the spermatic cord may be involved. In the residual testis, seemingly intact seminiferous tubules, even at a distance from the neoplasm, may be filled and expanded by seminomatous elements (Fig. 3). These probably represent early stages of neoplastic growth. The histologic pattern of the metastases is usually that of the seminoma from which it stems, but occasionally it simulates choriocarcinoma or embryonal carcinoma. This may indicate that the original neoplasm was of mixed cytologic content or that the metastatic epithelium had a multipotential germ cell quality and thus formed another tumor pattern. The presence of glycogen may be helpful in distinguishing this tumor from spermatocytic seminoma,

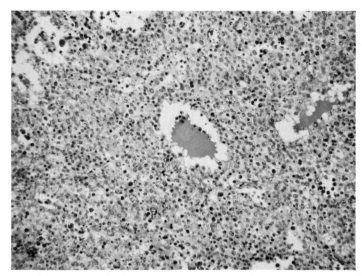

FIGURE 5.   Photomicrograph of a spermatocytic seminoma shows a tumor composed of germinal cells of variable size with the medium sized cells predominating. A lake of eosinophilic precipitate is present. (Hematoxylin and eosin; reduced from ×160).

lymphomas, or granulocytic sarcoma. Lymphoma may also be distinguished by exhibiting a strongly positive methyl green pyronine reaction. Granulocytic sarcomas often contain eosinophilic myelocytes and the granulocytic tumors show a positive napthyl-ASD-chloracetate stain (Leder stain).[10]

The anaplastic seminoma is more aggressive and has a poorer prognosis than classic seminoma.[11] In about 10% of seminomas the bulk of the tumor appears anaplastic.[1] The nuclei may be larger, more vesicular and irregular than in the typical seminoma, but increased mitotic activity is the most important and easily recognizable feature (Fig. 4). The diagnosis of anaplastic seminoma can be made where an average of three or more mitotic figures per high power field is found.[1] It is important to distinguish anaplastic seminoma from solid embryonal carcinoma. The cells of anaplastic seminoma are smaller, and less cohesive, and have more distinctive cellular borders than those of solid embryonal carcinoma.

Spermatocytic seminoma, originally described by Masson,[12] differs clinically, grossly, and microscopically from typical and anaplastic seminoma. Spermatocytic seminoma occurs exclusively in the testis and has not been associated with teratomatous elements.[13] It occurs most commonly over the age of 40 and comprises 9% of seminomas.[1] On gross examination the tumor tends to be softer, more gelatinous, and yellow. The microscopic appearance is characterized by three types of cells which differ distinctly in size (Fig. 5). The main cell type consists of medium-sized cells with a round nucleus and considerable eosinophilic cytoplasm. Intermixed with these cells are small cells and giant cells, which are usually mononuclear. The nuclei of the large cells have a filamentous or "spireme-like"

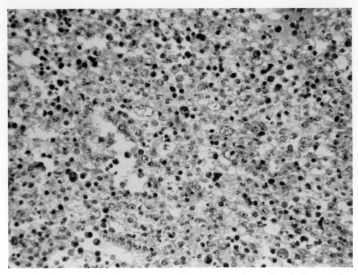

FIGURE 6. Photomicrograph of a spermatocytic seminoma shows that the large cells resemble primary spermatocytes in appearance. The small cells may represent degenerating forms. (Hematoxylin and eosin; reduced from ×250).

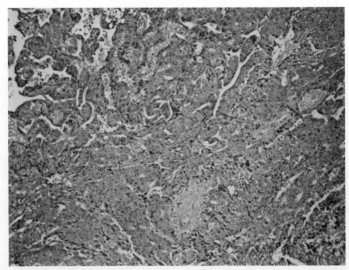

FIGURE 7. Photomicrograph of an embryonal carcinoma of the testis shows a predominantly solid tumor composed of large cells with a primitive epithelial appearance forming clefts and spaces (Hematoxylin and eosin; reduced from ×100).

chromatin distribution, similar to the meiotic phase of normal primary spermatocytes, which differentiates this tumor from other seminomas (Fig. 6). The
tumor cells usually occur in sheets and occasionally contain lakes of an eosinophilic
precipitate. The cytoplasm of the tumor cells is devoid of glycogen.[14] The stroma
is scant, and lymphocytic and granulomatous reactions are absent.[14] The spermatocytic type of seminoma is a differentiated tumor, which contains cells which
mimic spermatocytes of the normal seminiferous tubules; this tumor has a more
favorable prognosis than the classic seminoma.[13,15]

Embryonal Carcinoma

Embryonal carcinoma constitutes 15–20% of testicular neoplasms and usually
appears as a much smaller tumor than seminoma.[9] The affected testis is asym-
metrically enlarged, and the cut surface of the tumor has a gray or gray-red
heterogeneous appearance. Areas of hemorrhage and necrosis are common, but
gross cystic degeneration is absent. We believe the criteria for the recognition
of embryonal carcinoma of the testis, whether the patient is a child or an adult,
should be as specific as those used in the recent recognition of embryonal carcinoma of the ovary.[16,17] The tumor is composed of large, polygonal or ovoid cells
that have a primitive epithelial appearance, often with clear cytoplasm, growing
in a variety of patterns. The tumor may be made up of solid aggregates of cells,
or they may line clefts and spaces and form papillae (Fig. 7). True glandular
formations are not prominent. The cells have abundant pale eosinophilic granular
cytoplasm with indistinct cytoplasmic borders, frequently forming a syncytial
arrangement. The cells frequently overlap each other.[18,19] Nuclei are large and
centrally located, and often are pleomorphic, vesicular, and contain multiple
nucleoli. Mitotic figures, hemorrhage, and necrosis are common. The stroma may
have a cellular sarcomatous appearance, although this is rare in metastatic lesions.
The tumor metastasizes early to regional lymph nodes, where the histologic
pattern of the primary site may or may not be reproduced. The presence of
primitive neoplastic mesenchyme in some tumors does not justify the diagnosis
of an associated teratoma. Likewise, the presence of syncytiotrophoblastic giant
cells in an embryonal carcinoma should be noted, but the diagnosis of choriocarcinoma should not be made unless specific features of that tumor are
present.[1]

The cells of embryonal carcinoma usually contain abundant glycogen, best
demonstrated by using the periodic acid-Schiff technique prior to and after
diastase digestion.

The solid form of embryonal carcinoma must be distinguished from seminoma.
The lobular pattern of seminoma and the lymphocytic stroma are usually not
seen in embryonal carcinoma. The cells of embryonal carcinoma are usually
larger, more epithelial appearing, and more pleomorphic than those of seminoma.
In embryonal carcinoma mitoses are more frequent, cell membranes are less

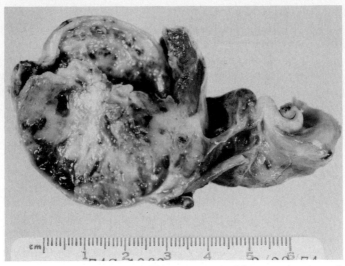

FIGURE 8.   Gross photograph shows a yolk sac carcinoma of the testis of a 14-month-old boy. The parenchyma is replaced predominantly by solid tumor with cystic and hemorrhagic areas.

distinct, and nuclei overlap. Well-prepared sections of properly fixed material are necessary to distinguish embryonal carcinoma from anaplastic seminoma.

Yolk Sac Carcinoma (Endodermal Sinus Tumor)

Yolk sac carcinoma of the testis was once considered a rare tumor of infancy and childhood. Teilum[20] recognized the similarity of this tumor to the endodermal sinuses of the rodent placenta, and termed it endodermal sinus tumor. Pierce, *et al.*[21] compared this tumor to a similar tumor of the mouse, and considered it to be a yolk sac or vitelline tumor. The tumors have been described under a variety of terms including testicular adenocarcinoma with clear cells occurring in infancy, distinctive adenocarcinoma of the infant's testis, orchidoblastoma, embryonal carcinoma of infants and children, embryonal carcinoma of the prepubertal testis, and infantile embryonal carcinoma. Talerman[22] found that testicular neoplasms commonly exhibit this histologic pattern in adults usually associated with one or more of the other germ cell tumors. Yolk sac elements were found in 38% of nonseminomatous germ cell tumors in adults, and in 10% of the cases were the predominant element.[22] Our own experience confirms these important observations. No pure yolk sac tumors in adults were encountered in his study, or in our own material.[23]

The gross appearance of this tumor is similar to that of embryonal carcinoma (Fig. 8). Yolk sac carcinomas exhibit a variety of histologic patterns, none of which is known to have prognostic significance. Five principal patterns have been described.[7,17]

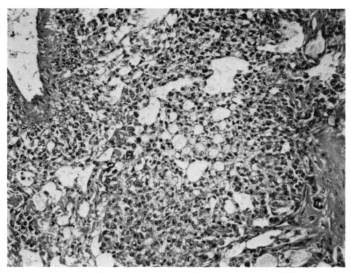

FIGURE 9.   Photomicrograph shows an area of yolk sac carcinoma exhibiting a microcystic pattern in a mixed germ cell tumor of the testis that occurred in a 33-year-old man. (Hematoxylin and eosin; reduced from ×100).

1. The microcystic and myxomatous pattern consists of a loose, vacuolated network, with small cystic spaces forming a honeycomb pattern (Fig. 9). The microcysts are lined by flat, pleomorphic, mesothelial-like cells that show frequent mitoses. The stroma has a loose myxomatous appearance considered to be analogous to the magma reticulare or extraembryonic mesoderm of the exocelom.

2. The endodermal sinus pattern is composed of perivascular formations consisting of a central capillary surrounded by a zone of connective tissue covered by a layer of cuboidal or low columnar epithelial cells (Fig. 10). The surrounding capsular sinusoidal space is lined by a single layer of flattened cells with hyperchromatic nuclei. These typical structures also known as Schiller-Duval bodies recapitulate the so-called endodermal sinus in the rat placenta. Such structures are not, however, conspicuous in the human placenta.

3. The solid cellular pattern is composed of aggregates of small epithelial-like polygonal cells with clear cytoplasm and frequent mitoses.

4. The alveolar glandular or cystic pattern is composed of alveoli, glandlike or cystic spaces lined by flat or cuboidal epithelial-like cells and surrounded by a myxomatous stroma or cellular aggregates.

5. The polyvesicular vitelline pattern has been described only in ovarian tumors and is composed of numerous cysts or vesicles surrounded by compact connective tissue stroma. The vesicles are lined partly by columnar or cuboidal cells and partly by flattened mesothelial-like cells. The wall of the cyst may show a constriction separating the parts lined by the different types of epithelium. This is considered to reflect the embryologic conversion of the primary yolk sac into the

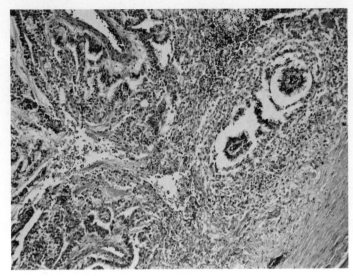

FIGURE 10.   Photomicrograph of an area of the same tumor as shown in Figure 9 shows an endodermal sinus pattern. Two Schiller-Duval bodies are seen on cross section on the right and another is shown in longitudinal section in the lower left. (Hematoxylin and eosin; reduced from ×100).

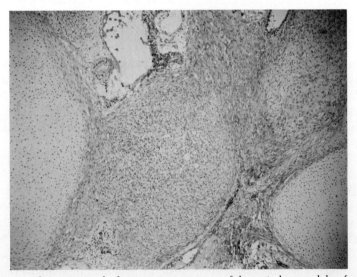

FIGURE 11.   Photomicrograph of an immature teratoma of the testis shows nodules of cartilage on each side and nodules of proliferating immature mesenchyme. Two small embryonic appearing glands are present in the upper part of the field. (Hematoxylin and eosin; reduced from ×63).

secondary yolk sac. Occasionally the whole tumor may exhibit the polyvesicular vitelline pattern. Such tumors have been referred to as polyvesicular vitelline tumors, and may have a favorable prognosis.

Small eosinophilic, PAS-positive diastase resistant globules may be present, either within tumor cells or outside them, and in some tumors they are numerous. These globules are considered to be secreted by the tumor cells and to accumulate in the cytoplasm. A similar material may be observed forming hyaline bands along the basement membrane. The latter deposits are considered to be analogous to Reichert's membrane of the mouse embryo.[24] These globules and the associated hyaline material can be shown immunocytochemically to contain alpha-feto-protein, alpha$_1$-antitrypsin, and basement-membrane-like material.

Yolk sac carcinoma must be distinguished from embryonal carcinoma, which has been considered to be more common in adults. Testicular tumors in adults formerly classified as embryonal carcinoma may have to be reinterpreted in terms of recent studies.[22] Embryonal carcinoma lacks the specific patterns observed in the endodermal sinus tumor. The tumor cells of embryonal carcinoma are frequently larger than those seen in the solid cellular aggregates in endodermal sinus tumor, the cytoplasm is more granular, there is more marked cellular and nuclear pleomorphism, and the nucleoli are more prominent.

Polyembryoma

Polyembryoma as defined by the World Health Organization is a tumor composed primarily of embryoid bodies.[3] The latter are structures containing a disc and cavities surrounded by loose mesenchyme simulating an embryo of about 2-weeks gestation. Endodermlike tubular structures and syncytiotrophoblast may also be present. Polyembryomas, as such, are extremely rare, but embryoid bodies are found more often within embryonal carcinomas or teratomas.

Choriocarcinoma

Choriocarcinoma is a highly malignant tumor composed of elements identical to syncytiotrophoblast and cytotrophoblast. Pure choriocarcinoma of the testis is extremely rare.[1] On the other hand, islands of choriocarcinoma are not uncommon in the other testicular neoplasms where the prognosis is not altered unless a large part of the lesion is replaced.

Pure choriocarcinoma is often quite small when detected but nonetheless may have metastasized widely. The tumor is often hemorrhagic and only a small rim of viable neoplasm may remain, the bulk of the tumor being necrotic. Essential to the histologic diagnosis is the existence of two distinct cellular components: large, cuboidal, or polyhedral clear cells with round or ovoid centrally placed nuclei in which the chromatin is coarse and clumped—the cytotrophoblast; and large pleomorphic, distorted cells with opaque eosinophilic cytoplasm and dark-staining, irregular nuclei either pyknotic or composed of coarse, vacuolated, and bubbly chromatin with giant, multiple nucleoli—the syncytiotrophoblast. These counterparts of placental elements may occasionally form pseudovilli. The syncytiotrophoblast usually comprises the advancing edge and is found eroding and invading blood vessels; for this reason massive hemorrhage is a frequent occurrence in both primary and secondary sites.

Teratoma

Testicular teratoma is a complex neoplasm containing recognizable elements derived from two or more germ layers. The involved testis is only moderately enlarged and section of the tumor reveals a gray-white honeycombed and cystic surface. Focally there may be cartilage, bone, and cystic cavities filled with either sebaceous material or clear serous fluid. On microscopic examination, ectodermal components often appear as stratified squamous epithelial-lined cysts and neural elements. The endoderm is represented by mucus-secreting glands and structures resembling gastrointestinal, respiratory, or urinary tracts. Mesodermal elements appear as cartilage, bone, muscle, and lymphoid tissue. Pure teratomas make up approximately 10% of testicular tumors.

The components of the tumor may be mature or immature or a mixture of this in varying proportions (Fig. 11). Mature elements may be differentiated, ranging from benign appearing cells to tissues and organs. Immature elements consist of primitive neuroectodermal, endodermal, or mesodermal tissue. Most of these tumors appear histologically benign, especially when cystic; however, they cannot be completely regarded so, since in nearly 30% of cases metastasis occurs within 5 years. Rarely, an adenocarcinoma or an epidermoid carcinoma may develop within an epithelial component of a teratoma.[1] The treatment of teratoma is, in general, that used in embryonal carcinoma. The 5-year survival rate is 71%.[25] We are not aware of any study comparing the degree of immaturity with the biologic behavior such as has been done with ovarian[26–28] and sacrococcygeal teratomas.[29] Dermoid cysts, frequent in the ovary, are very rare in the testis. On gross examination, dermoid cysts may contain hair, sebaceous and keratohyaline material, teeth, and bony and cartilaginous tissue. The cyst wall consists of keratinizing stratified squamous epithelium and skin appendages. Metastasis from a pure dermoid cyst has not been observed.[1]

Lesions Considered as One-Sided Development within a Teratoma

Two rare lesions of the testis are generally included under the classification of teratoma: epidermoid cysts and carcinoids. It has been postulated that these lesions represent one-sided development of a teratoma. When they occur by themselves, these lesions should not be diagnosed as teratomas, monodermal or otherwise, but by their specific morphologic features. Since the definition of teratoma requires the presence of elements of at least two germ layers, their

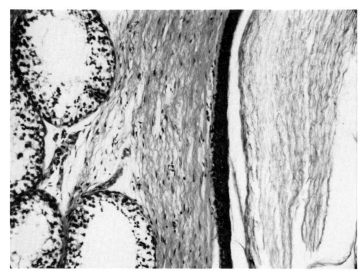

FIGURE 12.   Photomicrograph of testis shows seminiferous tubules to the left and a cyst lined by stratified squamous epithelium and containing laminated keratin to the right. (Hematoxylin and eosin; reduced from ×160).

histogenesis is unproven, and their biologic behavior differs markedly from the usual teratoma.

Simple Epidermoid Cyst

The simple epidermoid cyst is lined by keratinizing, stratified squamous epithelium supported by fibrous tissue (Fig. 12). The cyst is filled by keratohyaline material, and there are no skin appendages. About 1% of testicular tumors are simple epidermoid cysts. Price and Mostofi[30,31] reported that none of the 69 cases in the American Testicular Tumor Registry, including four in children, showed metastases when the tumor consisted only of a simple epidermoid cyst without scars or other elements. The majority of cases were discovered in the third decade of life.[30] This lesion should not be designated as teratoma because of the different prognostic implications of the latter term, but as an epidermoid cyst.

Carcinoid Tumor

Carcinoid tumor of the testis may be primary or metastatic.[1,32–35] It may be functional and give rise to symptoms of "carcinoid syndrome" upon palpation of the testis, or it may be nonfunctional and detected only as a testicular enlargement or nodule. Seventeen primary and six metastatic carcinoids in the testes have been reported.[33] Three of the primary tumors were associated with teratomas.[33] Primary testicular carcinoids are similar in appearance to ovarian car-

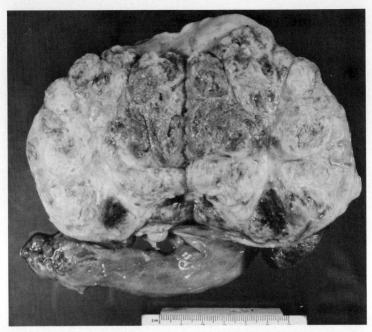

FIGURE 13.   Gross photograph shows the cut surface of a mixed germ cell tumor of the testis with areas of yolk sac carcinoma, seminoma, and immature teratoma (same case as Fig. 9). The tumor is solid and has a variegated appearance with extensive necrosis.

cinoids, have the typical appearances of carcinoids of midgut derivation by light and electron microscopy and the argentaffin reaction is positive.[33] The prognosis of primary testicular carcinoid is excellent; metastases have not been reported, but the prognosis of metastatic carcinoids to the testes is poor.[33]

Germ Cell Tumors Showing More than One Histologic Pattern

In about 40% of tumors of the testis, more than one histologic pattern is observed (Fig. 13). The occurrence of mixed patterns within germ cell tumors has caused much confusion in terminology.

Embryonal carcinoma and teratoma are most frequently associated; such a combination occurs in 24% of all testicular neoplasms.[1] Some authors have referred to this combination as teratocarcinoma. In addition to these components, seminoma is seen in 64% of the cases. Embryonal carcinoma and seminoma are seen in 5% of the cases. Almost any combination of germ cell tumor is possible, but no other specific combinations make up more than 3% of the cases. Although the term "teratocarcinoma" continues to be useful to clinicians, we agree with Mostofi and Price[1] that it is preferable for the pathologist to classify mixed germ cell tumors by naming the components. The term teratocarcinoma can be used in parenthesis where applicable.

One of the component types of tumor may be present in only a small focus, so careful examination of the gross specimen for areas that have a different appearance as well as the taking of many blocks of tissue is necessary for adequate histological sampling. In spite of these precautions, the metastases may be of different types from the primary tumor.

It is important to recognize the various combinations of germ cell tumors because the presence of a second component may influence clinical behavior, treatment, or prognosis in certain instances. Thus, Dixon and Moore[8] found the occurrence of seminoma in embryonal carcinoma and/or teratoma had no effect on the prognosis, but may affect the method of treatment. On the other hand, the prognosis of embryonal carcinoma is said to be ameliorated, if teratoma is present.[25] The presence of choriocarcinoma in significant amounts in an embryonal carcinoma or teratoma adversely affects the prognosis of the latter tumors.[1,8]

Mixed Germ Cell and Sex Cord-Stromal Tumor

Gonadoblastoma: Gonadoblastoma is a tumor containing both germ cells and sex cord-stromal elements.[36–38] These tumors may be interpreted as benign or in situ tumors, however, they have a marked tendency to be associated with germinomas. The gonadoblastoma develops in a dysgenetic gonad, either a streak gonad or a testis. These tumors occur in intersexes. Patients have actually been genetic males, i.e., they have a Y chromosome, usually with well-developed female characteristics. Microscopically, the tumor is composed of two principal cell types, large germ cells similar to those of seminoma and small cells resembling immature Sertoli and granulosa cells; elements resembling Leydig cells may also be present. Hyaline bodies are typically present. The tumor frequently shows calcification on microscopic examination.

Effect of Prior Chemotherapy

It must be understood by the pathologist examining specimens of germinal tumors after treatment of the patient by multiagent chemotherapy that profound effects will often be produced. Failure to recognize and interpret properly these changes may unnecessarily jeopardize relations with involved clinicians and potentially may have serious medico-legal consequences. Due to the extreme sensitivity of many of these tumors to present modalities of therapy, the tumor may be partly or completely destroyed. Thus, a retroperitoneal tumor mass considered by the clinicians to be a metastasis from a germinal tumor of the testis may be reduced to a mass of fibrous tissue containing numerous hemosiderin laden macrophages, or the pathologists may find similar foci in retroperitoneal

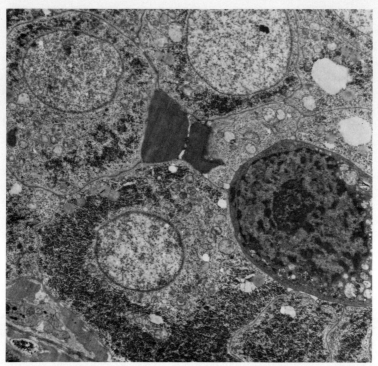

FIGURE 14.   Electron micrograph of seminoma. The tumor cells possess a low nuclear/cytoplasmic ratio. Note absence of membrane modifications. Observe large quantities of particulate glycogen within the cytoplasm. A lymphocyte is present on the right. (Lead citrate and uranyl acetate; reduced from ×5800).

lymph nodes. Although a positive diagnosis of malignancy cannot be made in such instances, the pathologist would do well to interpret such findings in light of the clinical history as being consistent with a nonviable treated tumor. Careful examination of the gross specimen to locate potentially viable areas and extensive sampling of grossly different appearing areas may be necessary to identify a small area of viable tumor in a large necrotic mass. The more mature the tumor tissue, the more likely it is to survive chemotherapy, so teratomatous elements appear relatively more common in specimens after treatment. We had seen one instance where the surgeon removed a tumor from the lung that had the appearance of mature teratoma in a patient with a primary embryonal carcinoma of the testis.

Immunocytochemistry

The recent application of immunofluorescent and immunoperoxidase techniques to testicular germinal neoplasms has provided important information

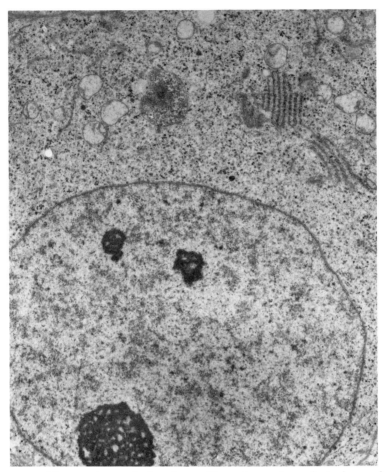

FIGURE 15.   Electron micrograph of seminoma. Observe large volume of cytoplasm and two stacks of granular endoplasmic reticulum. The nucleus has dispersed chromatin and multiple nucleoli. (Lead citrate and uranyl acetate; reduced from ×7500).

concerning the histogenesis of these neoplasms.[39] Teilum, Albrechtsen, and Nørgaard-Pedersen[40] demonstrated alpha-fetoprotein (AFP) within a testicular yolk sac carcinoma by immunofluorescent localization. More recently, Kurman, *et al.*[41] demonstrated AFP by an indirect immunoperoxidase technique in two of four testicular yolk sac carcinomas and seven of 15 adult embryonal carcinomas. It was localized to monodermal endodermal cells in all seven cases of the latter tumor and to hyaline droplets in four. In view of the fact that Talerman[22] has found yolk sac elements in 38% of adult germ cell tumors other than pure seminoma, and we have had a similar experience, we believe the presence of AFP may provide evidence of yolk sac elements. This viewpoint is strengthened by the fact that hyaline bodies were seen in four of these cases. Both AFP and alpha$_1$-antitrypsin have been identified in yolk sac carcinoma by the immunoperoxidase technique in five cases, two of which were testicular tumors.[42] In a case of ovarian yolk sac carcinoma, basement membrane antigen was demonstrated in hyaline globules and extracellularly.[43]

Human chorionic gonadotropin (HCG), considered characteristic of syncytiotrophoblast, was localized to trophoblastic giant cells of 12 of 15 embryonal carcinomas, but not to the mononuclear embryonal cells.[39] As would be expected, HCG was localized to syncytiotrophoblastic giant cells in two choriocarcinomas occurring as part of mixed germ cell tumors.[39] No localization of alpha-fetoprotein or HCG was noted in any case of seminoma or teratoma, with the exception that HCG was demonstrated in trophoblastic giant cells of a seminoma.[39]

In summary, AFP can be localized to yolk sac carcinomas, and also to some embryonal carcinomas in adults, where it may indicate the presence of yolk sac differentiation. HCG is localized to syncytiotrophoblastic cells whether they are a component of choriocarcinoma, or they occur as the syncytiotrophoblastic giant cells sometimes observed in other germ cell tumors.

Electron Microscopy

Introduction

The routine application of electron microscopy to the diagnosis of human neoplasms in the surgical pathology laboratory has increased remarkably in the past 5–10 years.[44-46] In general, fine structural study will objectively confirm a light microscopic impression or considerably narrow a histologic differential diagnosis.[46]

Within the testicular germ-cell tumor group, it is essential for therapeutic and prognostic reasons to clearly separate the seminoma-type neoplasms from the embryonal variants. Additionally, certain reticuloendothelial neoplasms, particularly large cell lymphoma, or metastatic carcinomas may simulate a primary germ cell tumor in both clinical presentation and pathologic appearance. Electron microscopic study, in most instances, will aid in resolving such diagnostic problems.

Seminomas

The fine structural features of the three types of seminoma have been described.[47-51] Classical and anaplastic seminomas are comparable except for minor quantitative differences.

The seminoma cell is large and polygonal with a low nuclear/cytoplasmic ratio (Fig. 14). The basal lamina, if present, is not conspicuous. Cell surface modifications, such as microvilli, are generally absent. Membrane contact specializations are simple and infrequent, consisting of small thickenings of apposed membranes.

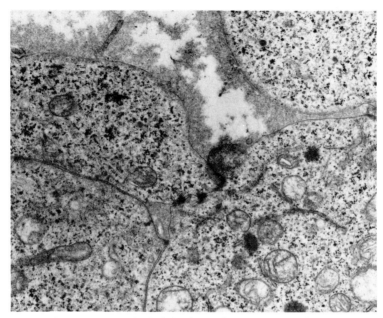

FIGURE 16.   Electron micrograph of solid embryonal carcinoma. Apically oriented tripartate junctional complexes are evidence of glandular differentiation. (Lead citrate and uranyl acetate; reduced from ×13,300).

The cytoplasm is distinguished by containing pools of particulate glycogen. The usual organelles are represented with occasional parallel stacks of ribosome bearing endoplasmic reticulum (Fig. 15). The Golgi complex may be well developed. Lysosomes are inconsistently present. Nuclear profiles are moderately indented with dispersed chromatin. Nucleoli display a consistent configuration of multiple skeinlike filaments, each associated with a pars amorpha.

Spermatocytic seminomas show more differentiation at the ultrastructural level than is evident in anaplastic and classic testicular seminoma.[51] Among the more distinctive differences are that the nuclei are more uniformly rounded than in the other forms of seminoma, and occasional filamentous structures resembling chromosomes in the leptotene stage of meiotic division are observed. Glycogen is inconspicuous. Characteristically, intercellular cytoplasmic bridges are occasionally seen in spermatocytic seminoma cells, similar to the bridges that occur between normal primary spermatocytes and spermatids.

Solid Embryonal Carcinoma

The ultrastructure of solid embryonal carcinoma has been studied considerably less than that of seminoma.[50] These cells are large and rounded also with a low nuclear/cytoplasmic ratio. In sharp contrast to seminoma, the basal lamina is

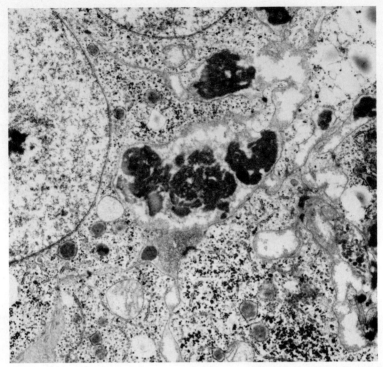

FIGURE 17.   Electron micrograph from area of yolk sac carcinoma (same case as Fig. 9) shows granular flocculent material within cisternae of granular endoplasmic reticulum as well as aggregates of similar material, which may represent early stages in the formation of the hyaline bodies seen by light microscopy. (Lead citrate and uranyl acetate; reduced from ×8500).

conspicuous, limiting groups of cells. Acinar formations of varying degrees of complexity are present. These are characterized by apically oriented junctional complexes (Fig. 16) associated with projecting microvilli. Mature desmosomes are frequent and are laterally oriented. The cytoplasmic organelles show a greater degree of development than observed in seminoma; the ribosome bearing endoplasmic reticulum and Golgi complexes may be highly developed. Secretory products, however, are generally not observed in solid embryonal carcinoma. Particulate glycogen may be observed, though with less consistency and in lesser quantity than observed in seminoma. Nuclear structure and configuration are often comparable to that of seminoma.

Yolk Sac Carcinoma (Endodermal Sinus Tumor)

We are not aware of reported ultrastructural studies of yolk sac carcinoma of the testis, but observations of a testicular mixed germ cell tumor with elements of yolk sac carcinoma, immature teratoma, and seminoma in a man and four other

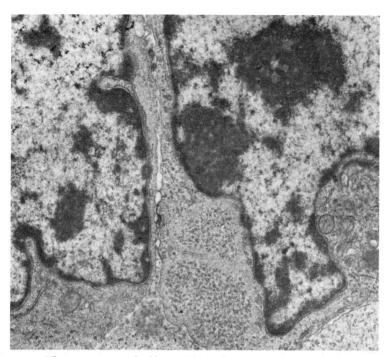

FIGURE 18.   Electron micrograph of large cell lymphoma. Note absence of cell contacts and membrane modification. The cytoplasm is dominated by polyribosome rosettes. (Lead citrate and uranyl acetate; reduced from ×16,250).

yolk sac tumors suggest that the ultrastructural appearance of the tumor, although somewhat variable, is independent of its site of occurrence.

The most characteristic feature of the tumor seems to be the presence of flocculent granular material of variable density within distended cisternae of granular endoplasmic reticulum, as well as the presence of similar material extracellularly[43,52] (Fig. 17). This material appears to be condensed intracellularly to form hyaline bodies. Another significant feature was the presence of abundant glycogen particles. The tumor nuclei were markedly irregular in shape, although uniform in size. In many nuclei there was a prominent threadlike nucleolonema similar to that described in germinoma cells. Where a group of tumor cells surrounded a lumen, numerous microvilli were present. Elsewhere, cells were either closely applied with frequent desmosomal attachments or were separated by extracellular electron dense material.

Large Cell Lymphoma

As mentioned earlier, reticuloendothelial neoplasms, particularly large cell lymphoma, may present as a testicular mass.[53–55] The histology of the neoplasms

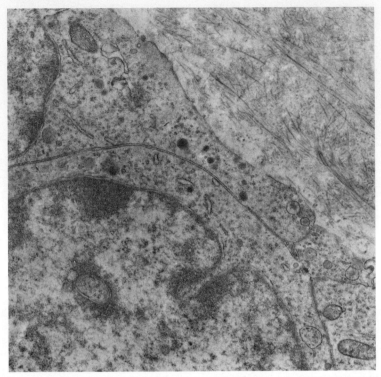

FIGURE 19.   Electron micrograph of metastatic oat cell carcinoma to the testis. Small membrane bound dense core granules are present within the cytoplasm. (Lead citrate and uranyl acetate; reduced from ×16,300).

may closely simulate that of anaplastic seminoma or solid embryonal carcinoma. The diagnostic ultrastructural features of large cell ("histiocytic") lymphoma have been described and appear to be comparable in all sites.[56-58] The tumor cells have been shown to represent large transformed lymphocytes, rather than to be of monocyte-macrophage origin.[59] Cell contact sites, membrane modifications, and basal lamina are consistently absent. The cytoplasm contains a monotonous and dense array of polyribosomes (Fig. 18); other organelles are inconspicuous. Glycogen is invariably absent. The chromatin is dispersed and one to two large, dense nucleoli are present.

Metastatic Carcinoma

Metastatic carcinoma involving the testes can simulate a primary testicular neoplasm clinically. We have seen a metastatic oat cell carcinoma involving the testis in which the primary lung tumor was not recognized initially, and orchiectomy was performed. Demonstration of neurosecretory granules within the cytoplasm of the tumor cells confirmed the diagnosis (Fig. 19).

Table IV.

	Seminoma	Solid embryonal carcinoma	Yolk sac carcinoma	Large cell lymphoma
Basal lamina	±; poorly developed	++; conspicuous	++; conspicuous	—
Microvilli	±; infrequent; poorly formed	++; frequent; well formed	++; frequent well formed	—
Cell contacts	+; infrequent; small desmosomes	++; frequent complex tripartate junctions; mature desmosomes	++; frequent complex tripartate junctions; mature desmosomes	—
Acinar formation	—	+	+	—
Organelles	Heterogeneous; moderately developed	Heterogeneous; highly developed	Heterogeneous; highly developed	Homogeneous; polyribosomes
Glycogen	++	±	+	—
Secretion granules	±; small lysosome	—	++; "hyaline bodies"	—

Summary of Ultrastructure

In summary, diagnostic electron microscopy can often clearly separate the seminomatous germ cell tumors from the nonseminoma types. The ultrastructure of yolk sac tumors appear to be characteristic. Large cell lymphoma or metastatic small cell carcinoma simulating a germ cell neoplasm are clearly distinguished at the fine structural level.

The ultrastructural diagnostic features of germ cell tumors are summarized in Table IV.

References

1. Mostofi, F. K., and Price, E. B., Jr.: Tumors of the male genital system. *Atlas of Tumor Pathology*, Fascicle 8, Series 2, Washington, D. C.: Armed Forces Institute of Pathology, 1973.

2. Friedman, N. B., and Moore, R. A.: Tumors of the testis: A report of 922 cases. *Milit Surg* **99:**573–593, 1946.

3. Mostofi, F. K., and Sobin, L. H.: *International Histologic Classification of Tumours, No. 16. Histological Typing of Testis Tumors.* Geneva: World Health Organization, 1977.

4. Willis, R. A.: Teratomas. *Atlas of Tumor Pathology*, Fascicle 9, Series 1. Washington, D. C.: Armed Forces Institute of Pathology, 1951.

5. Collins, D. H., and Pugh, R. C. B.: *The Pathology of Testicular Tumours.* Edinburgh and London: E. & S. Livingstone, Ltd., 1964.

6. Teilum, G.: Classification of endodermal sinus tumour (mesoblastoma vitellinum) and so-called "embryonal carcinoma" of the ovary. *Acta Pathol Microbiol Scand* **64**:407–429, 1965.

7. Teilum, G.: Special tumours of the ovary and testis. *Comparative Histology and Identification*, 2nd ed. Philadelphia: J. B. Lippincott Co., 1976.

8. Dixon, F. J., and Moore, R. A.: Tumors of the male sex organs. *Atlas of Tumor Pathology*, Fascicle 31b and 32, Series 1. Washington, D. C.: Armed Forces Institute of Pathology, 1952.

9. Mostofi, F. K., and Leetsma, J. E.: The genitourinary tract. *Concepts of Disease. A Textbook of Pathology*. Brunson, J. G., and Gall, E. A. (Eds.). New York: The MacMillan Company, 1971, pp. 756–790.

10. Leder, L. D.: Uber die selektive fermentcytochemische Darstellung von neutrophilen myeloischen Zellen und Gewebsmastzellen im Paraffinschnitt. *Klin Wochenschr* **42**:553, 1964.

11. Maier, J. G., Sulak, M. H., and Mittemeyer, B. T.: Seminoma of the testis: Analysis of treatment success and failure. *Am J Roentgenol* **102**:596–602, 1968.

12. Masson, P.: Étude sur le séminome. *Rev Can Biol* **5**:361–387, 1946.

13. Rosai, J., Silber, I., and Khodadoust, K.: Spermatic seminoma. I. Clinicopathologic study of six cases and review of the literature. Cancer **21**:92–102, 1969.

14. Scully, R. E.: Spermatocytic seminoma of the testis. A report of 3 cases and review of the literature. Cancer **14**:788–794, 1961.

15. Fox, J. E., and Abell, M. R.: Spermatocytic seminoma. *J Urol* **100**:757–761, 1968.

16. Kurman, R. J., and Norris, H. J.: Embryonal carcinoma of the ovary. A clinicopathologic entity distinct from endodermal sinus tumor resembling embryonal carcinoma of the adult testis. *Cancer* **38**:2420–2433, 1976.

17. Talerman, A.: Germ cell tumors of the ovary. *Pathology of the Female Genital Tract*. Blaustein, A. (Ed.). New York: Springer-Verlag 1977, pp. 527–585.

18. Nochomovitz, L. E., de la Torre, F. E., and Rosai, J.: Pathology of germ cell tumors of the testis. *Urol Clin North Am* **4**:359–378, 1977.

19. Nochomovitz, L. E., and Rosai, J.: Current concepts on the histogenesis, pathology and immunochemistry of germ cell tumors of the testis. *Pathol Annu* **13**:327–362, 1978. Part I.

20. Teilum, G.: Endodermal sinus tumors of the ovary and testis. Comparative morphogenesis of the so-called mesonephroma ovarii (Schiller) and extraembryonic (yolk sac-allantoic) structures of the rat's placenta. *Cancer* **12**:1092–1105, 1959.

21. Pierce, G. B., Bullock, W. K., and Huntington, R. W., Jr.: Yolk sac tumors of the testis. *Cancer* **25**:644–658, 1970.

22. Talerman, A.: The incidence of yolk sac tumor (endodermal sinus tumor) elements in germ cell tumors of the testis in adults. *Cancer* **36**:211–215, 1975.

23. Roth, L. M., and Panganiban, W. G.: Gonadal and extragonadal yolk sac carcinomas. A clinicopathologic study of 14 cases. *Cancer* **37**:812–820, 1976.

24. Pierce, G. B., Midgley, A. R., Jr., Feldman, J. D., Sri Ram, J., and Feldman, J. D.: Parietal yolk sac carcinoma: Clue to the histogenesis of Reichert's membrane of the mouse embryo. *Am J Pathol* **41**:549–566, 1962.

25. Mostofi, F. K.: Testicular tumors. Epidemiologic, etiologic and pathologic features. *Cancer* **32**:1186–1201, 1973.

26. Thurlbeck, W. M., and Scully, R. E.: Solid teratoma of the ovary. A clinicopathological analysis of 9 cases. *Cancer* **13**:804–811, 1960.

27. Norris, H. J., Zirkin, H. J., and Benson, W. L.: Immature (malignant) teratoma of the ovary. A clinical and pathologic study of 58 cases. *Cancer* **37**:2359–2372, 1976.

28. Nogales, F. F., Jr., Favara, B. E., Major, F. J., and Silverberg, S. G.: Immature teratoma of the ovary with a neural component ("solid" teratoma). A clinicopathologic study of 20 cases. *Hum Pathol* 7:625–642, 1976.

29. Gonzalez-Crussi, F., Winkler, R. F., and Mirkin, D. L.: Sacrococcygeal teratomas in infants and children. Relation of histology and prognosis in 40 cases. *Arch Pathol* 102:420–425, 1978.

30. Price, E. B., Jr.: Epidermoid cysts of the testis: A clinical and pathologic analysis of 69 cases from the Testicular Tumor Registry. *J Urol* 102:708–713, 1969.

31. Price, E. B., Jr., and Mostofi, F. K.: Epidermoid cysts of the testis in children: A report of four cases. *J Pediatr* 77:676–679, 1970.

32. Brown, N. J.: Miscellaneous tumours of epithelial type. *Pathology of the Testis*. Pugh, R. C. B. (Ed.). Oxford: Blackwell Scientific Publications, 1976, pp. 304–316.

33. Talerman, A., Gratama, S., Miranda, S., and Okagaki, T.: Primary carcinoid tumor of the testis: Case report, ultrastructure and review of the literature. *Cancer* 42:2696–2706, 1978.

34. Simon, H. B., McDonald, J. R., and Culp, O. S.: Argentaffin tumor (carcinoid) occurring in a benign cystic teratoma of the testicle. *J Urol* 72:892–894, 1954.

35. Kemble, J. V.: Argentaffin carcinomata of the testicle. *Br J Urol* 40:580–584, 1968.

36. Scully, R. E.: Gonadoblastoma. A gonadal tumor related to the dysgerminoma (seminoma) and capable of sex-hormone production. *Cancer* 6:445–463, 1953.

37. Scully, R. E.: Gonadoblastoma. A review of 74 cases. *Cancer* 25:1340–1356, 1970.

38. Talerman, A., and Delemarre, J. F. M.: Gonadoblastoma associated with embryonal carcinoma in an anatomically normal man. *J Urol* 113:355–359, 1975.

39. Taylor, C. R., Kurman, R. J., and Warner, N. E.: The potential value of immunohistologic techniques in the classification of ovarian and testicular tumors. *Hum Pathol* 9:417–427, 1978.

40. Teilum, G., Albrechtsen, R., and Nørgaard-Pedersen, B.: Immunofluorescent localization of alpha-fetoprotein synthesis in endodermal sinus tumor (yolk sac tumor). *Acta Pathol Microbiol Scand* (A) 82:586–588, 1974.

41. Kurman, R. J., Scardino, P. T., McIntire, K. R., Waldmann, T. A., and Javadpour, N.: Cellular localization of alpha-fetoprotein and human chorionic gonadotropin in germ cell tumors of the testis using an indirect immunoperoxidase technique. A new approach to classification utilizing tumor markers. *Cancer* 40:2136–2151, 1977.

42. Palmer, H. E., Safaii, H., and Wolfe, H. J.: Alpha₁-antitrypsin and alpha-fetoprotein. Protein markers in endodermal sinus (yolk sac) tumors. *Am J Clin Pathol* 65:575–582, 1976.

43. Nogales-Fernandez, F., Silverberg, S. G., Bloustein, P. A., Martinez-Hernandez, A., and Pierce, G. B.: Yolk sac carcinoma (endodermal sinus tumor). Ultrastructure and histogenesis of gonadal and extragonadal tumors in comparison with normal human yolk sac. *Cancer* 39:1462–1474, 1977.

44. Bonikos, D. S., Bensch, K. G., and Kempson, R. L.: The contribution of electron microscopy to the differential diagnosis of tumors. *Beitr Path Bd* 158:417–444, 1976.

45. Györkey, F., Min, K. W., Kuisko, I., and Györkey, P.: The usefulness of electron microscopy in the diagnosis of human tumors. *Hum Pathol* 6:421–441, 1975.

46. Mackay, B. and Osborne, B. M.: The contribution of electron microscopy to the diagnosis of tumors. *Pathobiol Annu* 8:359–405, 1978.

47. Holstein, A. F., and Körner, F.: Light and electron microscopic analysis of cell types in human seminoma. *Virchows Arch* (A) *Pathol Anat* 363:97–112, 1974.

48. Janssen, M. and Johnston, W. H.: Anaplastic seminoma of the testis. Ultrastructural analysis of three cases. *Cancer* 41:538–544, 1978.

49. Levine, G. D.: Primary thymic seminoma. A neoplasm ultrastructurally similar to testicular seminoma and distinct from epithelial thymoma. *Cancer* 31:729–741, 1973.

50. Pierce, G. B., Jr.: Ultrastructure of human testicular tumors. *Cancer* 19:1963–1983, 1966.

51. Rosai, J., Khodadoust, K., and Silber, I.: Spermatocytic seminoma. II. Ultrastructural study. Cancer 24:103–116, 1969.

52. Gonzalez-Crussi, F., and Roth, L. M.: The human yolk sac and yolk sac carcinoma. *Hum Pathol* 7:675–691, 1976.

53. Givler, R. L.: Testicular involvement in leukemia and lymphoma. *Cancer* 23:1290–1295, 1969.

54. Silvert, M. A., and Gray, C. P.: Reticulum cell sarcoma of testis. *Urology* 4:395–399, 1976.

55. Woolley, P. V., III, Osborne, C. K., Levi, J. A., Wiernik, P. H., and Canellos, G. P.: Extranodal presentation of non-Hodgkin's lymphomas in the testsis. *Cancer* 38:1026–1035, 1976.

56. Gillespie, J. J.: The ultrastructural diagnosis of diffuse large-cell ("histiocytic") lymphoma. Fine structural study of 30 cases. *Am J Surg Pathol* 2:9–20, 1978.

57. Glick, A. D., Leech, J. H., Waldron, J. A., Flexner, J. M., Horn, R. G., and Collins, R. D.: Malignant lymphomas of follicular center cell origin in man. II. Ultrastructural and cytochemical studies. *J Natl Cancer Inst* 54:23–36, 1975.

58. Levine, G. D., and Dorfman, R. F.: Nodular lymphoma. An ultrastructural study of its relationship to germinal centers and a correlation of light and electron microscopic findings. *Cancer* 35:148–164, 1975.

59. Lukes, R. J., and Collins, R. D.: A functional classification of the malignant lymphomas. *The Reticuloendothelial System*, International Academy of Pathology Monograph. Baltimore: Williams and Wilkins Co., 1975, pp. 213–242.

2

Surgical Management of Testis Cancer

John P. Donohue, M.D.

Urology Department, Indiana University Medical Center, Indianapolis, Indiana

I. Initial Diagnosis and Radical Orchiectomy

Initial Diagnosis

INITIAL DIAGNOSIS IS the key to therapy. Greater than 50% of testis cancer is misdiagnosed as epididymitis initially. Delays of effective treatment during antibiotic trials are reported in every major series. There is a great public health need for lay teaching of scrotal exam. Testis cancer is the most common solid tumor in men between the ages of 15 and 40 (2.1–2.3 per 100,000). If local teaching at every medical school and hospital level regarding scrotal exam is intensified, earlier diagnosis will be likely greeted with lower stage lesions on clinical presentation. As it stands now, in our series, less than ⅓ of our patients are Stage A. The others have advanced metastatic disease, and most were misdiagnosed as "epididymitis" on their initial presentation. Therefore, this medical center has begun a visual aid program using 2 × 2 carousels depicting appropriate exam and, also, development of silastic teaching models for scrotal exam. The critical feature of scrotal exam is the digital separation of the intrascrotal contents. The testis presenting anteriorly can be separated from the adnexal epididymal and cord structures posteriorly quite simply by insinuating the thumb and forefingers between them and then sliding the testis incased in the firm tunica

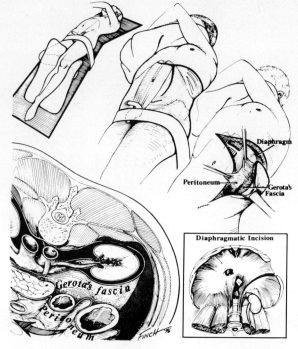

FIGURE 1A. Position of patient for retroperitoneal lymphadenectomy via thoracoabdominal approach, modified T-square incision suggested by Fraley.[3]

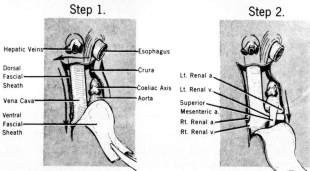

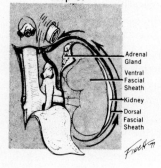

FIGURE 1B. First three steps as outlined by Fraley.[3]

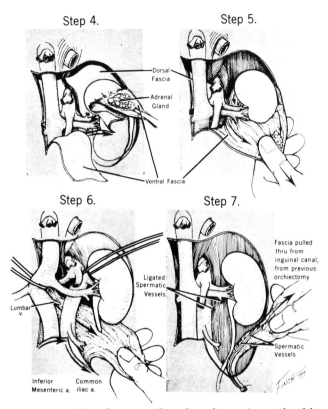

FIGURE 1C. . Next four steps (four through seven) as outlined by Fraley for retroperitoneal lymphadenectomy via thoracoabdominal approach.[3]

albuginea back and forth between the thumb and forefingers. Any solid mass within the testis can easily be palpated in this manner. Public acceptance of male self-examination (analogous to acceptance of female self-exam of the breast) will follow provided the physicians at every level of medicine promote this principle of male self-exam. The Indiana experience suggests not only the need; but the great increase in early referrals here in the last several years suggests the efficacy of this program.

Orchiectomy

Any time a scrotal mass is felt to be a possible testis tumor, inguinal approach is mandatory. The inguinal cord is clamped and preferably divided before the tunics are stretched and the testis expressed into the wound. This prior clamping is to prevent tumor emboli via the cord which can be promoted by tumor manipulation. Turnbull's work of the "no touch" technique in handling tumors has been confirmed experimentally.[1] Manipulation of tumors is shown to produce lymphatic and, at times, venous tumor emboli. Another important preoperative consideration is the understanding on the patient's part that the testis is an expendable organ. Consent needs to be signed for total orchiectomy even if the physician is uncertain of the nature of the mass. Words like "exploration" and "biopsy" are mentioned only to be condemned. The patient should be clearly advised that the tumor should be removed for excisional biopsy ex vivo by the pathologist.

A word about technique of orchiectomy. Inguinal incision is made and the external oblique fascia divided over the presumed level of the internal ring, and then the internal oblique muscle is either separated in the direction of its fibers or divided. Then the inguinal cord can be visualized lying on the transversalis fascia below. This is picked up and divided into its vascular and vasal components which then are doubly clamped and divided. We recommend double ligatures proximally. Then the internal ring is dilated and the vasal and vascular segments of the cord stump can be pushed into the retroperitoneal space to facilitate future spermatic vein removal at the subsequent retroperitoneal lymphadenectomy, should this be required. The inverted scrotal attachments to the testis and epididymis (gubernaculum) can then be divided between clamps or with electrocautery. Meticulous hemostatis is necessary. No drain is used in the scrotum as a rule.

If the scrotum is contaminated by prior biopsy of tumor in situ, then hemiscrotectomy and inguinal lymphadenectomy will be required owing to proclivity of tumor implant in the scrotal tunics. Preferably, this can be done as a separate procedure. Often, following retroperitoneal lymphadenectomy which will determine the Stage A vs. B, the inguinal lymphadenectomy and hemiscrotectomy can be done within several weeks. We recommend that this not be done in conjunction with retroperitoneal lymphadenectomy. The relative increased incidence of suppuration in scrotal wounds suggests it is wiser to separate these two procedures lest the larger retroperitoneal wound be contaminated. Johnson and Babaian[21] quite rightly question the routine application of inguinal or iliac lymphadenectomy in all cases of scrotal orchiectomy. In 19 such cases only three (19%) had local scrotal recurrence. None had inguinal lymphadenectomy nor subsequent nodal disease in that area. Treatment was hemiscrotectomy alone. A reasonable view would be to reserve inguinal nodal surgery only for those with clear wound tumor spillage at surgery (e.g., tumor biopsy in situ) who have considerable delay (several weeks) between contamination and subsequent hemiscrotectomy, obvious scrotal disease, or suspicious inguinal adenopathy. Otherwise, the yield of positive inguinal nodes is so low in cases of scrotal orchiectomy as to not warrant the routine application of extended inguinal lymphadenectomy in all cases of scrotal orchiectomy.

II. Radical Retroperitoneal Lymphadenectomy for Staging and Treatment

A. Thoracoabdominal

The thoracoabdominal approach to retroperitoneal lymphadenectomy has been well described by Leadbetter[2] and, more recently, by Fraley[3] and Skinner.[4]

Advantages of this approach are ease of exposure of the ipsilateral hilar and suprahilar region, an opportunity to palpate the ipsilateral lower lung and resect nodule(s) if necessary, and less postoperative ileus if the extraperitoneal approach is employed. Disadvantages are difficulty in doing bilateral dissection, especially in the contralateral suprahilar region, poor iliac bilateral exposure, and time of wound opening and closing.

The reader is referred to these good descriptions for further detail on the thoracoabdominal technique. Several illustrations of both thoracoabdominal and transabdominal approaches are included in this monograph.

B. Transabdominal

The rationale and technique of the anterior approach for retroperiotoneal lymphadenectomy for the purpose of staging nonseminomatous germinal cell tumors of the testis have been well described by Patton and Mallis[5] and Van-Buskirk and Young[6] and, more recently, by both Staubitz, et al.[7,8] and Whitmore.[9] Also, Young[10] described this approach in one of the more recent standard urology texts.

An alternative approach to the retroperitoneum for staging testicular tumors by lymphadenectomy was championed by Leadbetter.[2] He preferred the thoracoabdominal approach, which affords exposure above the renal hila. This approach has been followed, with some modifications, by Fraley, et al.[3] and Skinner[4] with great success.

Twelve years ago we asked ourselves, "Can the midline approach also be developed to allow excellent exposure of the suprarenal hilar zones for the purpose of lymphadenectomy?" Postmortem dissections of the retroperitoneum were done through a midline incision from xiphoid to pubis to determine whether this approach could equal the high exposure afforded by the thoracoabdominal approach. As of this writing, more than 150 patients with nonseminomatous germinal tumors of the testis have been staged by high retroperitoneal lymphadenectomy through the anterior approach, using the techniques herein described, to afford optimum exposure and nodal clearance.

Special Preoperative Preparation and Medical Notes. These patients are prepared, as a donor for renal transplantation would be, with overnight intravenous hydration. We use no antibiotics preoperatively or postoperatively.

The bladder is catheterized at the time of draping in surgery. The catheter is usually removed on the second postoperative day. The patient is in the supine position with the right arm suspended from an ether screen or with both arms extended. Mannitol, 12.5–25 g, is given intravenously during the first part of the operation to prevent the oliguria attendant on extensive bilateral renovascular dissections. Topical 1% xylocaine or Papaverine 30 mg/cc is used on the renal vessels during the dissection. Emphasis is placed on the intraoperative administration of colloid to replace large third space losses of lymph during the dissection. Otherwise, falsely high misleading hematocrit values may follow. An increased need for crystalloid also is apparent as the losses from the intravascular space into the large, raw third space created in the retroperitoneum can produce significant contractions of effective blood volume. Often transfusions of whole blood are unnecessary in uncomplicated cases if enough colloid replacement is given.

Preoperative emphasis on pulmonary physiotherapy is given in order to assist the patient postoperatively in this regard. Again, no prophylactic antibiotics are used. If fever develops, appropriate cultures and investigations are made, and then the drug is selected; but this is rarely necessary.

Technique. Exposure: The incision is midline, xiphoid to pubis. Drapes are sewn in place and an 11-in. circular plastic wound protector is used, then two Balfour abdominal retractors are placed. The abdomen is explored carefully by palpation. Then the basic mesenteric divisions are made in order to mobilize the entire small bowel and right colon so that they can be placed on the patient's chest in a plastic bowel bag. First, the hepatic flexure is taken down, and then the mesocolon is incised from the foramen of Winslow to the cecum. It is important to extend this posterior peritoneal incision through the base of the foramen of Winslow, which covers the anterior surface of the vena cava, because later dissection must extend above this area.

After the right mesocolon is divided, the incision is turned around, and the root of the small bowel is incised cephalad to the ligament of Treitz. This incision is carried along the root of the bowel until the inferior mesenteric vein is encountered. This vein must be divided in order to carry the incision in an oblique manner further cephalad, still further into the left upper quadrant, paralleling the inferior border of the pancreas. If the inferior mesenteric vein is not divided, it will restrict the exposure in this area. When the inferior mesenteric vein is divided, the pancreas can be mobilized fully and retracted off the anterior surface of Gerota's fascia. Then the anterior surface of Gerota's fascia is separated bluntly and sharply from the undersurface of the bowel and the pancreatic head and body, as well as the duodenum and cecum. All of this is now completely mobilized. A routine appendectomy is done, and the bowel is placed on the chest in a bowel bag.

Suprarenal Hilar Dissection. The dissection is started at the superior mesenteric artery. The head and the body of the pancreas are elevated by two deep Harrington retractors after they are covered with a laparotomy pad. The left colic mesentery has been separated from Gerota's fascia and retracted laterally. This

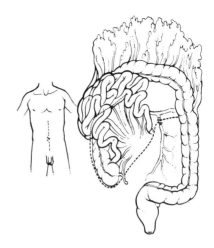

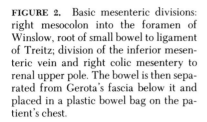

FIGURE 2. Basic mesenteric divisions: right mesocolon into the foramen of Winslow, root of small bowel to ligament of Treitz; division of the inferior mesenteric vein and right colic mesentery to renal upper pole. The bowel is then separated from Gerota's fascia below it and placed in a plastic bowel bag on the patient's chest.

separation of the left colic mesentery is later continued inferiorly and facilitated by dividing the inferior mesenteric artery so as to enhance the exposure of the middle and inferior retroperitoneal space. When the head of the pancreas is elevated in broad Harrington or Dever retractors, the superior mesenteric artery is further exposed. The splanchnic nerves are divided between clips, as are the lymphatics from around the superior mesenteric artery. The dissection is carried down around the aorta and cephalad between the aorta and either crus of the diaphragm. Ganglia and lymphatics are clipped and divided on either crus. The dissection continues cephalad below the Harrington reactors, and the tissue is drawn down and doubly clipped and divided as high as possible at the base of the diaphragm. Just above this, between the aorta and the vena cava, is the base of the cisterna chyli.

The right suprahilar dissection is then continued across the crus of the diaphragm to the medial aspect of the inferior vena cava (Fig. 2). This vessel is then further dissected in the subadventitial plane by the right adrenal gland between vascular clips. Then the dissection is carried down to the renal vessels. The adventitia of the renal artery and vein is divided. The dissection is carried out to the right renal hilum just beyond the bifurcation of the renal vessels. This bloc of nodal and ganglionic tissue is then dissected off the posterior body wall, sharply, between vascular clips. In years past, this tissue was rotated below the renal vessels and kept en bloc with the infrahilar aortocaval package of nodes. In recent years we have been submitting this tissue separately for analysis in order to determine how many nodes there are usually in the right suprahilar zone. The usual range is from four to eight.

The left suprahilar dissection is accomplished by dividing the left adrenal vein as it enters the renal vein and splitting the adventitia of the renal vein and carrying this out to the left renal hilum and up medial to the adrenal gland (Fig. 3). Clipping along the medial aspect of the adrenal gland and rotating and elevating

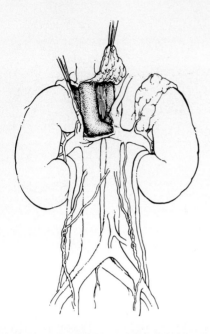

FIGURE 3. The right suprahilar dissection extends up the aorta from the superior mesenteric artery, onto the crus of diaphragm, over to the medial aspect of the right adrenal gland about 4–6 cm above the right renal artery, then down the medial border of the right adrenal gland to the right renal artery, and along the renal artery back to the aorta.

it out of the way exposes the renal hilum, the fat pad, and the nodal tissue medial to the kidney. Then, by blunt and sharp dissection, the tissue is mobilized off the posterior body wall. Also, the dissection on the aorta between the crura is carried cephalad obliquely about 4–6 cm above the left renal artery. Nodal tissue between the aorta and the body wall and the foramen of L1-L2 is an important and constant drainage point from the nodes just inferior to this at the left renal hilum. The several adrenal arterial branches from the aorta and the proximal left renal artery are divided between clips. Nodal and ganglionic tissue is peeled off the posterior body wall and, again, rotated either dorsal or ventral to the left renal artery from which it is mobilized by sharp dissection in the subadventitial plane. This tissue is submitted separately as the left suprarenal hilar package. The usual number of nodes here is four to 10.

Infrarenal Hilar Dissection (Aortocaval Dissection). This portion of the procedure has been well described in several communications. Basically, the nodal package is split anteriorly down over the inferior vena cava and aorta. The specimen is then rotated off the vessels. This author believes that it is important to divide every lumbar vessel, both aortic and caval, so as to get complete mobilization and central vascular control. Another important maneuver is the squaring out of the upper corners of the nodal package at each renal hilum and taking it down off the posterior body wall at the foramen of L2-L3 (Figs. 4 and 5). The lateral borders of the dissection are the ureters; the psoas fascia is stripped down parallel to this. The gonadal vein is divided on the left from the renal vein or on the right from the inferior vena cava. The involved gonadal vein is then followed

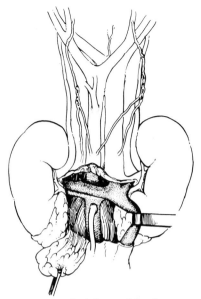

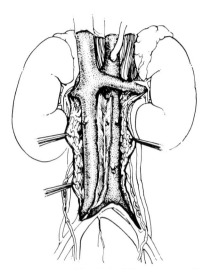

FIGURE 4. The left suprahilar dissection extends from the superior mesenteric artery up the left side of the aorta, onto the crus and up 4–6 cm above the left renal artery. The left renal vein and artery are mobilized caudad, the adrenal vein is divided, and the adrenal gland is rotated cephalad after all its medial attachments are divided between clips. The tissue is taken off the crus and foramina by sharp dissection between clips.

FIGURE 5. The infrahilar aortocaval dissection involves the anterior longitudinal splitting of the nodal and vascular adventitia over the vena cava and aorta, its lateral rotation, and the "squaring out" of the nodal package at each renal hilum at the renal vessels. Every lumbar vessel is divided to facilitate en bloc removal of posterolateral nodal tissue.

down to its origin in the groin and dissected out separately and submitted to the pathologist separately.

Care is taken to obtain the divided stump of the spermatic cord with its original ligatures if at all possible. The vas deferens is clipped and divided so that the distal portion can be submitted with the spermatic vein and cord stump. On the left side this is then tunneled under the left colic mesentery. The aortic dissection is continued distally by dividing the inferior mesenteric artery. The left colic mesentery is then further mobilized off Gerota's fascia, and the splanchnic nervous and venous connections are clipped where necessary to mobilize this thoroughly and hence expose the iliac areas from the medial approach without having to divide the left mesocolon. The left ureter is then easily seen over the pelvic brim. As noted earlier, the nodal packages are rotated off the anterior surfaces of both vessels, the dissection being advanced in the sub-adventitial planes. This allows easy exposure of each lumbar artery and vein and their division between 2–0 silk ligatures. Now the great vessels are completely mobilized (Figs. 6 and

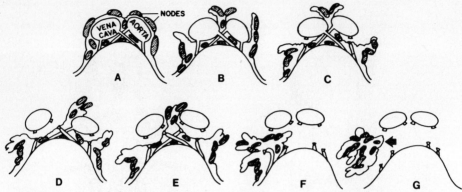

FIGURE 6.   An axial view showing the anterior split of the nodal package in the subadventitial plane (B) and its rotation off the vena cava and aorta after the division of each lumbar vessel (C–E). Then the specimen is removed from the posterior body wall by ligating and sharply dividing all the lumbar vessels and ganglia as they emerge from the foramina. The specimen is easily rotated under the mobilized great vessels after these posterior attachments are divided.

7). The only thing holding the unfurled nodal package is its posterior and lateral attachments.

Each lumbar artery and venous penetration into the posterior body wall is divided between clips or ligatures. Bleeding venous tributaries are often controlled by Bovie coagulation or additional suture ligature (Fig. 7). Once the posterior attachments are divided at the foramina, the nodal package can be wiped off the anterior spinous ligaments with a gauze sponge and drawn under the vessels either medially or laterally. Again, it is convenient for our nodal analysis to submit the aortocaval package of nodes separately and then later to submit the two iliac dissections separately. Formerly, the entire specimen was obtained en bloc and

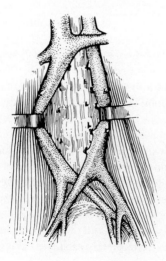

FIGURE 7.   At the conclusion of the dissection, the anterior spinous ligaments and medial psoas muscle are seen stripped bare. The lumbar vessels are tied off on the body wall as well as on the great vessels. Each foramen is clear of nodal tissue. Fully mobilized great vessels allow thorough inspection.

laid out on a predrawn template for the pathologist. There were some errors in nodal location once the tissue was placed in formalin because, occasionally, the tissue would float off the paper template.

The iliac dissections extend several centimeters beyond the bifurcation of the hypogastric artery on either side. The same principal of nodal rotation beneath the vessels is employed. The anterior division of the arteries and veins is carried out, and the tissue is rotated below these after the division of any lumbar attachments. It is important to mobilize the psoas muscle in retractors because the nodal chain in the paravertebral area here is often large but not clearly visible without mobilization of the psoas. Again, the right iliac and left iliac nodal packages are submitted separately.

The wound is then thoroughly inspected and irrigated. When tumor invasion of the nodes is grossly evident, we irrigate with warm distilled water, which might lyse any tumor cells that may have been spilled in the wound during dissection. Then we close the mesenteric attachment with running 00 chromic catgut beginning at the left posterior colonic mesentery to the left upper quadrant and proceeding below the pancreas to the ligament of Treitz. Closure is then carried down, closing the root of the small bowel to the cecum. After this, the right mesocolon is closed from the cecum up to the foramen of Winslow. We believe that this helps to prevent postoperative bowel complications and that it limits the escape of bloody lymphatic fluid into the peritoneal cavity. The omentum is drawn down over the bowel. The position of the Levin tube is checked. The midline incision is closed with interrupted 0 Prolene sutures placed in the manner of Jones. Buried knots are tied below the fascia to avoid uncomfortable nodules in the subcutaneous tissue in thin patients. Number 2 Merselene retention sutures are used in patients with grossly tumorous nodes whom we know will have chemotherapy in several weeks, with some resultant delay in wound healing and increased abdominal pressure due to the vomiting caused by chemotherapy.

Results. At the time of this writing, more than 150 patients have been staged with retroperitoneal lymphadenectomy as just described. Crude 3-year survival rates are available for these patients.

All of our 55 patients with Stage A disease continue to survive. Their management was simple. After a thorough staging lymphadenectomy, if the nodes contained no tumor, the patients were monitored by monthly chest radiographs for the first year, every other month for the second year, every third month for the third year, etc. In recent years we have begun testing every 1 month for the beta subunit of human chorionic gonadotropin and for alpha fetoprotein. Of the 55 patients with Stage A disease followed from 2 to 12 years who were so treated, five developed Stage C disease with pulmonary metastases (9%). All five continue to survive with no evidence of disease. One patient was treated with intravenous Actinomycin-D and local chest radiotherapy 8 years ago. A lobectomy after this treatment revealed no persistent tumor. The other four patients have been treated with combination chemotherapy consisting of Cis-platinum, Velban, and

Bleomycin. They are in complete remission, with no evidence of tumor, and all patients have been off maintenance chemoprophylaxis for 2 years.

Fifty patients were classified as having Stage B disease with nodal involvement in the retroperitoneum; 45 of these 50 (90%) survive, all clinically tumor free. Most of these patients were treated with adjuvant Actinomycin-D 1 mg intravenously every day for 4 consecutive days at monthly intervals for 12–24 months. However, since 1976, most of the Stage B patients were treated with no adjuvant chemotherapy. There did not appear to be any obvious benefit in the relapse rate for those patients who received adjuvant Actinomycin-D. An integral part of the postoperative management is monthly chest radiographs and serum HCG and alphafetoprotein for the first year after surgery, and every other month the second postoperative year.

Therefore, 100 of our 105 patients with Stage A or Stage B disease survive, all clinically tumor free, for a cumulative survival rate of 95% in these two stages. Since July 1973, the advent of our use of combination chemotherpay (AVB of PVB) for relapsing Stage B patients, 95% of our Stage B patients (37 of 39) are living and well with no evidence of disease 2–5 years post node dissection.

In addition to the staging retroperitoneal lymphadenectomies, we have performed retroperitoneal operations on 26 patients with Stage C disease that were coverted to Stage B disease with chemotherapy. When the patient's chest had cleared, and there was still evidence of persistent retroperitoneal disease, surgical removal was accomplished. Twenty-two of these 26 patients survive, and all are clinically in complete remission.

This brings us to the next surgical area for testis cancer, namely, cytoreductive surgery.

III. Cytoreductive Surgery

Special consideration should be given to cytoreductive surgery for testis cancer.

Several years ago it was felt primary cytoreductive surgery of massive metastatic tumors would reduce "tumor burden" for subsequent chemotherapy. Hence, dramatic efforts were made to debulk patients of large retroperitoneal tumors and even multiple pulmonary lesions. One such series[11] reported encouraging survival of 43% despite significant surgical morbidity. A theoretical and actual problem with this approach was the need for aggressive chemotherapy in the postoperative patient, often immunosuppressed by his massive disease. Occasionally, needed chemotherapy was delayed by virtue of surgical complications.

The advent of cell cycle drugs with much higher cell kill ratios when used in effective combinations allowed consideration of *chemical* rather than surgical cytoreduction. This has proven to be roughly twice as effective as earlier primary surgical cytoreduction. The method usually used with chemical cytoreduction

Table I.

Combination Chemotherapy Followed by Cytoreductive Surgery Patient Survival

Indiana	UCLA
22/26	20/24

involves treating the patient with multiple metastases with drug combinations such as Platinum, Velban, and Bleomycin for a series of four courses for 3–4 months. Once the patient demonstrates resolution of pulmonary metastases and reduction of retroperitoneal tumor mass, which many do, then secondary surgical cytoreduction becomes more feasible. Residual retroperitoneal tissue is resected. About one-third of the cases will have persistent testis cancer, another one-third will have mature teratoma differentiation, and the final third will have fibrous or cystic tissue only, having been cleared of all tumor by their chemotherapy. This approach seems more effective; it gives the patient with disseminated disease what he needs first, namely systemic chemotherapy. It also puts surgery in a more elective framework.

The results speak in favor of primary chemical cytoreduction followed by *secondary* surgical resection. Two such series[13,4] report survival in excess of 80% in patients pretreated with chemotherapy prior to surgical resection (Table I).

Also commentary regarding technique of secondary cytoreductive surgery is in order. There is the question of how much to resect. Should only the residual "lump" of tissue be excised or should the dissection include all of the retroperitoneal area once occupied by nodal tissue draining the testis? There is no perfect knowledge here. This author prefers the latter choice, viz., a whole dissection because it is a more complete, representative sample of the retroperitoneal tissue which may have once been involved with tumor. Peeling this fibrous, desmoplastic tissue off the great vessels can be tedious and difficult. At this point one might argue it would be easier to do multiple biopsies only. The problem with this approach is apparent. Are such random biopsies representative of all the retroperitoneal nodal tissue? Experienced surgeons recall instances when relatively innocent-looking gross tissue contained microscopic tumor. To avoid this pitfall, this author recommends as complete a dissection as possible even in these secondary cases.

IV. Miscellaneous Surgical Procedures

A. Hemiscrotectomy

A contaminated scrotum is said to occur when a testicle was biopsied in situ and tumor discovered. Also, transcrotal approach to orchiectomy when questioning tumor preoperatively is to be condemned. Tumor cells spilling in scrotal tissue take the lymphatic drainage pathways to the ipsilateral superficial inguinal nodes. Hence, in cases of potential scrotal contamination not only a hemiscrotectomy but also an ipsilateral superficial inguinal lymph node dissection is recommended in cases where there is nodal enlargement or delayed referral.

While high inguinal approach to the suspected testis tumor seems common knowledge to urologic surgeons, many operations for scrotal problems are still done by generalists. Twenty-one of 64 patients referred to University of Minnesota hospitals from 1964 to 1974 had contaminated scrotums from inadequate initial approaches, including needle aspiration, transcrotal biopsy, and transcrotal orchiectomy.

A good description by Markland[13] considers more fully the management considerations in such cases. The recent report of Johnson[21] mentioned earlier suggests an alternative conservative approach to the inguinal area.

B. Thoracotomy

Thoracotomy is occasionally necessary for tissue diagnosis of a persistent pulmonary lesion following chemotherapy. Rarely, some initial tomograms show a solitary lesion that is questioned as possible granuloma. Before beginning chemotherapy, thoractomy, and nodule resection can be done. But this is not often necessary as other methods (markers, CAT scans, fiberoptic transbronchial biopsies, or needle aspiration biopsies, etc.) usually can be employed to discriminate tumor vs. granuloma in equivocal cases.

Commentary

Our position is that the more thorough the lymphadenectomy, the more accurate the staging. The merits of a bilateral dissection vs. a unilateral dissection remain debatable. The report by Ray, et al.[14] of their standard infrahilar dissections indicates that contralateral spread is rare in the face of tumor-free ipsilateral nodes. Perhaps one purpose of the unilateral dissection was to preserve ejaculation. It appears, however, that the majority of patients are still unable to ejaculate even after this form of dissection according to reports by Johnson[15] and others. Also, the fact that contralateral spread sometimes occurs, particularly in the face of ipsilateral nodal involvement with tumor, suggests the merit of a thorough bilateral dissection.

The merits of a suprahilar dissection in combination with the standard hilar and infrahilar approach are still less well known. Admittedly, it is rare that a patient would have disease in the suprahilar nodes in face of tumor free infrahilar nodes (it happened in only two of our first 60 patients). But it is not rare to have the suprahilar nodes involved when the infrahilar nodes contain tumor. In our series, one of every four patients with tumor-containing infrahilar nodes also had tumor in the suprahilar nodes. Several of our patients with tumorous suprahilar nodes had apparently tumor-free nodes at the time of dissection and were found

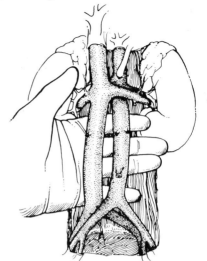

FIGURE 8. The aorta and the inferior vena cava can be manipulated easily during and after the dissection when all the lumbar vessels and the inferior mesenteric artery have been divided. Hemostasis is easily secured with this exposure and vascular mobility. Complete clearance of nodes and removal of bulky tumor deposits are achieved better with this central vascular control.

to have microscopic involvement of their suprahilar nodes as well as their infrahilar nodes. It seems reasonable then to clear out the nodal drainage pathways of the testis completely if we are to stage and treat with surgery as thoroughly as possible.

A disadvantage of the suprahilar extended approach through the midline is that it does take longer than the standard hilar and infrahilar approach. A minimum of $1\frac{1}{2}$ hr is added to the time of this procedure so that the total operating time averages 5–6 hr in an uncomplicated case.

Questions are often asked about the value of total vascular mobilization by dividing all the lumbar vessels. In our series there have been no spinal cord complications from this procedure. Ferguson, *et al.*,[16] in a literature review, reported 28 cases of paraparesis following total infrarenal aortic replacement for aneurysm in older males. But this study relates to an older group of patients who had lost their primary anterior descending spinal blood supply because of atherosclerotic cardiovascular disease in the thoracic aorta and its branches, and who had been depending on their lumbar arteries for collateral circulation. In our younger patients this is not a problem. We believe that vascular mobilization is necessary because lateral views and dissection studies have shown that there are as many nodes and lymphatics behind the great vessels and posterolateral to them as there are above them. Also, the lymphatics occupy each lumbar foramen, and there are many tumor-containing nodes found in these foramina in patients with Stage B disease.

It is a fact that the best results in the last decade in the management of patients with testicular tumors are to be found in those medical centers in which the surgical staff is committed to a thorough retroperitoneal lymphadenectomy.[17,18,3] Those authors espousing a partial and less aggressive lymphadenectomy do not have the data to support their contention that such limitation provides a superior method of staging and treatment.

Still another area of controversy that should be mentioned concerns the role of radiotherapy in the management of these patients. In brief, it can be said that the need for radiotherapy is contracting sharply in the face of great advances in chemotherapy. In our experience,[17] radiotherapy was a negative factor if the patients developed Stage C disease, as all Stage B patients are at risk of doing. The impact of prior radiotherapy on the bone marrow is lasting. More persistent and profound luekopenia in patients treated earlier with radiotherapy limits the chemotherapist in his ability to deliver effective doses of chemotherapy. Eight of our nine deaths were related to complications of radiotherapy, either directly or indirectly. This finding will form the basis of a separate report.

Summary

In summary, several conclusions can be drawn from our experience. Chemotherapy is opening new avenues in the management of these patients. It allows us to leave patients with Stage A disease untreated, with close follow-up. Should Stage C disease develop, the patient can be salvaged with appropriate and aggressive combination chemotherapy, as our cases were. Patients with Stage A disease should have a 100% survival rate if the retroperitoneum is dissected appropriately and the patient is followed closely postoperatively. Several options exist for the postoperative management of patients with Stage B disease. Three courses are under cooperative study: (a) no treatment, as in Stage A; (b) one-drug chemoprophylaxis with Actinomycin D; and (c) combination chemotherapy from the onset. We have treated Stage B cases with Actinomycin D therapy from 1965 to 1975. Those patients who developed Stage C disease have been switched to combined chemotherapy with Cis-Platinum, Velban, and Bleomycin. Since 1974, all of our patients with Stage B disease who progressed to Stage C have achieved complete remission with this three-drug combination. Another new horizon is the potential for chemical cytoreduction of disseminated Stage C disease; persistent abdominal disease can then be resected. It is this author's opinion that chemotherapy provides a safer, more extensive initial cytoreduction than the contrary approach of primary surgical cytoreduction and postoperative chemotherapy.

Sero testing for the beta subunit of human chorionic gonadotropin and for alpha fetoprotein has been a helpful means of following patients with Stage B disease and for detecting tumor before it can be seen by any of the conventional radiologic methods.[19,20]

Although the future of retroperitoneal lymphadenectomy is still unclear and improvements in noninvasive staging will doubtless continue (sero testing for tumor associated antigens, ultrasound, axial tomography, and lymphangiography), it would seem doubtful that highly accurate staging can be obtained without surgical dissection and histologic nodal examination. We and others[18] have noted that as many as one-third of our patients in whom all these preoperative tests for metastases (including sero testing) were negative, nonetheless had evidence of multiple tumorous nodes on microscopic examination. This suggests that the role of surgical staging with histologic nodal study will remain central to the accurate definition of the disease status and further direction of therapy. Furthermore, retroperitoneal surgery, completely done, seems to have positive influence on patient survival in this disease.

References

1. Turnbull, R. B., Kyle, K., Watson, F. R., and Spratt, J.: Cancer of the colon: The influence of the no-touch isolation technic on survival rates. *Cancer* 18(2): 82–87, 1968.

2. Skinner, D. G., and Leadbetter, W. F.: The surgical management of testis tumors. *J Urol* 106:84–93, 1971.

3. Fraley, E., Markland, C., and Lange, P.: Surgical treatment of Stage I and Stage II non-seminomatous testicular cancer in adults. *Urol Clin North Am* 4(3):453–463, 1977.

4. Skinner, D. G.: Management of non-seminomatous tumors of the testis. *Genitourinary Cancer.* Skinner and deKernion (Eds.). Philadelphia: W. B. Saunders, 1978, pp. 470–493.

5. Patton, J. F., and Mallis, N.: Tumors of the testis. *J Urol* 81:457–461, 1959.

6. VanBuskirk, K. E., and Young, J. G.: The evolution of the bilateral antegrade retroperitoneal lymph node dissection in the treatment of testicular tumors. *Milit Med:* July 1948.

7. Staubitz, W. J., Magoos, I. V., Grace, J. T., and Shenk, W. G., III: Surgical management of testis tumors. *J Urol* 100:350, 1969.

8. Staubitz, W. J., Early, K. S., Magoos, I. V., and Murphy, G. P.: Surgical treatment of non-seminomatous germial testis tumors. *Cancer* 32:1206, 1973.

9. Whitmore, W. F., Jr.: Treating germinal tumors of the adult testes. *Contemp Surg* 6:17, 1975.

10. Young, J. D., Jr.: Retroperitoneal surgery. *Urologic Surgery,* 2nd ed New York: Harper & Row, pp. 848–857.

11. Merrin, C., Takita, H., Beckley, S. and Kassis, J.: Treatment of recurrent and widespread testicular tumors by radical reductive surgery and multiple sequential chemotherapy. *J Urol* 117:291–295, 1977.

12. Donohue, J. P. and Einhorn, L.: The timing and place of cytoreductive surgery for extensive testis cancer. Submitted for publication. *J Urol:* May 1979.

13. Markland, C.: Special problems in managing patients with testicular cancer. *Urol Clin North* Am 4(3):427–449, 1977.

14. Ray, B., Hajou, S. I., and Whitmore, W. F.: Distribution of retroperitoneal lymph node metastases in testicular germinal tumors. *Cancer* 33:340, 1974.

15. Johnson, D. E.: Testicular Turmors. 2nd ed., Med. Exam. Publ. Co., 1976. Personal communication.

16. Ferguson, L. R. J., Bergan, J. J., and Conn, J., Jr., *et al.*: Spinal ischemia following abdominal aortic surgery. *Ann Surg* 181:267, 1975.

17. Donohue, J. P., Einhorn, L. H., and Perez, J. M.: Improved management of non-seminomatous testis tumors. *Cancer* 42:2903–2908, 1978.

18. Skinner, D. G., and Scardino, P. T.: Relevance of biochemical tumor markers and lymphadenectomy in management of non-seminomatous testis tumors: Current perspective. Submitted for publication. *J Urol:* March 1979.

19. Javadpour, N.: The national cancer institute experience with testis cancer. *J Urol* **120:** 651–659, 1978.

20. Lange, P. H., McIntire, K. R., Waldmann, T. A., Hakala, T. R., and Fraley, E. E.: Serum alpha fetoprotein and human chorionic gonadotropin the in diagnosis and management of non-seminomatous germ cell testicular cancer. *N Engl J Med* **295:**1237, 1976.

21. Johnson, D. E., and Babaian, R. J.: The case for conservative surgical management of the ilioinguinal region after inadequate orchiectomy. Submitted for publication, *J Urol*.

3

The Role of Radiation Therapy in the Management of Adult Germinal Testis Tumors

William U. Shipley, M.D.

Massachusetts General Hospital, Harvard Medical School, Boston, Massachusetts

Introduction

SURGERY BY RADICAL INGUINAL ORCHIECTOMY is both the appropriate diagnostic step and the treatment of choice for the control of the primary site of a patient with testicular tumor.[1,2,19] Radiation therapy by megavoltage external beam irradiation is one of the treatment options for the control of the regional lymph node metastases. The rationale for the use of radiation therapy or surgery to treat the regional (retroperitoneal) lymph node metastases in the curative management of patients with testicular tumors is that at presentation a substantial number of patients, depending on histology, will have metastases only to the retroperitoneal lymph nodes. Thus, control of the disease at this first site of metastasis by local treatment, either radiation therapy or surgery, will lead to cure in this group of patients with testicular cancer.

Table I.
Radiation Therapy in Testicular Seminoma

Institution	Clinical Stage I		Clinical Stage II	
	Number	% 3-year disease-free survival	Number	% 3-year disease-free survival
Walter Reed[5]	284	97%	34	76%
Royal Marsden Hospital[6]	78	98%	27	93%
M. D. Anderson Hospital[4]	79	94%	30	74%
Stanford University[7]	71	100%	27	89%
Rotterdam Institute[8]	91	100%	46	91%
Total	603	97%	164	85%

Pure seminoma, the most common subtype of testicular tumors,* is the most radiosensitive malignancy managed in radiotherapy clinics, although solid leukemic deposits may be of almost equal radiosensitivity. Both can nearly always be sterilized by doses of 2000–3000 rad with conventional fractionation.[4] Because of the exquisite radiation sensitivity of seminomatous deposits, radiation therapy, rather than surgical resection, is the treatment of choice to the retroperitoneal lymph nodes for patients presenting with this germ cell tumor. As will be discussed below, the 3-year disease-free survival results of radiation therapy following radical orchiectomy in patients with Stage I or II testicular seminoma are 97% and 85% respectively in the 767 patients reviewed (Table I). This extraordinarily high success rate makes seminoma to date surpassed only by skin cancer as the most successfully managed group of tumors in all of oncologic clinical practice.

Lymph node metastasis from nonseminomatous germ cell tumors of the testis (histologic Groups II–V of Dixon and Moore), while clearly less sensitive than seminoma (*vide infra*) are still, relative to epithelial cancers, quite radiation sensitive—about similar to that of Hodgkin's disease. For instance, the local cure rate following 4500 rads with conventional fractionation for small to moderate-sized lymph node metastases (Stage IIA)† from nonseminomatous testis cancer is 93%,[12] which is comparable to the 95% reported in Hodgkin's disease.[13]

---

* Dixon and Moore Classification[3] of germ cell testicular tumors. Group I: pure seminoma; Group II: embryonal carcinoma, pure or with seminoma; Group III: teratoma, pure or with seminoma; Group IV: teratoma with embryonal and/or choriocarcinoma, with or without seminoma; Group V: Choriocarcinoma, pure or with embryonal carcinoma and/or seminoma.

† Clinical staging of testicular carcinoma, presented both by Maier and Lee[9] and Peckham[10] based on their experience and that of the M. D. Anderson Hospital.[11] Clinical Stage I: Lymphangiogram negative, no evidence of metastases; Clinical Stage IIA: Lymphangiogram positive with maximum diameter of metastases less than 2cm, evidence of metastases confined to retroperitoneal nodes; Clinical Stage IIB: Lymphangiogram positive with maximum diameter of metastases 2cm or greater, evidence of metastases confined to retroperitoneal nodes; Clinical Stage III: Involvement of supra- and infra-diaphragmatic lymph nodes, no evidence of extralymphatic metastases; Clinical Stage IV: Extralymphatic metastasis.

Understanding the clinical similarities (and the differences) of these testis cancers to Hodgkin's disease, which has had both effective chemotherapy and radiation therapy for more than a decade, is helpful in a critical review of the best present therapeutic strategies of combining surgery, radiation therapy, and chemotherapy most effectively. Germinal cell testicular cancers are similar to Hodgkin's disease in that: 1) they occur in a relatively young population in which considerations of cure and cure with maintenance of fertility are important; 2) both diseases have an orderly spread with systemic dissemination occurring only infrequently when patients have no or minimal metastatic disease to the first echelon (testis cancer) or contiguous (Hodgkin's disease) lymph nodal region; 3) moderately extensive regional lymph node disease is quite sensitive to well tolerated doses of external beam radiation therapy; 4) effective multidrug chemotherapy is now available yielding a significant probability of cure in patients presenting with extranodal disease; and 5) lymphangiography is 70%–80% accurate in both types of malignancy but clearly a less exact staging procedure than surgical sampling; thus, in either testis cancer or Hodgkin's disease the treatment results of all series must be evaluated in light of the method by which the patients were staged because such differences in staging, rather than differences in treatment, may explain the possible differences in results. Of course, despite these remarkable clinical similarities germinal cell tumors of the testicle are histologically totally distinct from Hodgkin's disease and thus differ in many respects. Some differences that influence the planning of therapeutic strategies are: 1) the primary testicular tumor is well managed surgically such that in only unusual circumstances is radiation therapy to the primary site necessary; 2) the recent development of detectable serum markers by radioimmunoassay (human chorionic gonadotrophin, HCG, and alpha-feto protein, AFP) has improved staging accuracy in patients with nonseminomatous testicular tumors;[14] and 3) the usual surgical approach to the retroperitoneal nodes in testis cancer, but not in Hodgkin's disease, has been a radical dissection with *both* diagnostic and therapeutic intent.

While the role of radiation therapy in the treatment of seminoma and Hodgkin's disease is well established, the role of radiation therapy in the treatment of patients with nonseminomatous germ cell testicular carcinoma is less clear. As will be reviewed, surgical lymph node resections, external beam radiation therapy, or multidrug chemotherapy all are effective modes of treating patients with minimal (or no detectable) regional lymph node metastases. Therefore, the selection of modality, of the combination of modalities, is best done with an understanding not only of the efficacy of each of these therapies, but the potential harmful sequellae that may result from such treatments. The comparative efficacy of radiation in the management of patients with nonseminomatous testicular cancer is presented in detail in this chapter. Based on this analysis (*vide infra*), the author thinks that the treatment of choice following radical orchiectomy for patients with nonseminomatous testicular cancer to be: 1) for clinical Stage I disease—external beam radiation therapy (4500 rads) to the retroperitoneal lymph nodes; 2) for clinical Stage IIA disease—preoperative radiation therapy (3000 rad) combined with a modified lymph node dissection and adjuvant chemotherapy only in patients with histologically proven residual nodal metastases; and 3) for clinical Stages IIB, III, and IV disease—primary multidrug chemotherapy with either surgery and/or radiation therapy used for residual disease.

Treatment Techniques

Clinical Evaluation

Prior to final treatment recommendations several important postorchiectomy evaluations must be at hand. All the slides of the radical orchiectomy specimen must be reviewed by an experienced pathologist. In our experience this has led to an altered diagnosis in the type of germinal cell testicular tumor in approximately 20% of patients referred. While this may seem surprisingly high, I believe it is understandable when one realizes how relatively infrequently a general pathologist in a community hospital is called upon to diagnose these uncommon tumors. The important discrimination by the pathologist is pure seminoma vs. nonseminomatous malignant lesions. The clinical staging for the evaluation of possible extragonadal metastatic disease should always include whole lung tomograms, bipedal lymphangiogram, and quantitative pre- and postorchiectomy serum radioimmunoassay of HCG and AFP. These, with the possible assistance of the retroperitoneal CT scan, are all necessary for accurate clinical staging of the patient prior to the final recommendation for therapy to the potentially involved retroperitoneal lymph nodes. Bipedal lymphangiography has an accuracy of 70%–80% when compared to pathologic staging as reported from many large centers.[15-19] However, the accuracy of clinical (lymphangiographic) staging for the detection of retroperitoneal lymph nodes is improved further by the additional evaluation of postorchiectomy serum markers. In a recent review of the Memorial Sloan Kettering Cancer Center experience, 86% or 32 of 37 patients found to have metastases on retroperitoneal node dissection had a positive lymphangiogram and/or an elevated serum HCG or AFP.[14]

Radiation Techniques

Lymphangiographic visualization of the retroperitoneal lymph nodes is essential in the careful design of the appropriate retroperitoneal treatment field with radiation therapy. Exact definition of field extent depends on the details for a given patient and the type of megavoltage equipment utilized. Figure 1 demonstrates radiotherapeutic fields usually employed for patients with Clinical Stage I or IIA testicular cancer. As the lymphatic drainage differs for the left and right testicles, so should the field in the region of the renal hila depending on the side of the tumor involvement. Generally these contoured anterior and posterior fields extend *superiorly* to the origin of the thoracic duct or to include the anterior

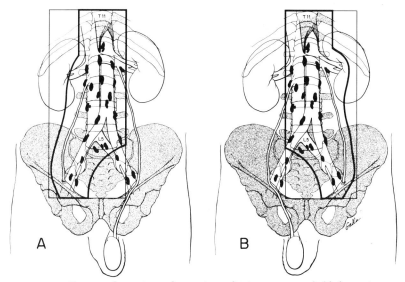

FIGURE 1. Contoured anterior and posterior radiation treatment fields for patients with clinical Stage I or IIA testicular cancer but without epididymal involvement or prior inguinal surgery. A right testicular tumor; B left testicular tumor.

surface of T11 vertebral body and *inferiorly* to the ipsilateral inguinal region. The inferior margin is not extended below the inguinal ligament unless there has been a history of prior inguinal or scrotal surgery that may predispose to atypical lymphatic drainage. Laterally, the margins should include the *ipsilateral* renal hilum, usually more generous on the left than on the right, and the *contralateral* retroperitoneal lymph nodes of the para-aortic or paracaval and common iliac groups. If there has been evidence of epididymal invasion by the tumor, the fields should be enlarged to include the ipsilateral hypogastric lymph node group as a potential site of metastastic drainage. Note these fields are only slightly more encompassing than those of a modified bilateral surgical dissection.[17,19] While some institutions prefer to treat the ipsilateral external iliac and inguinal lymph nodes with a separate anterior field, we have found with the use of secondary cerroband blocking of our 10-MV linear accelerator fields these areas can be very satisfactorily treated in continuity. Excretory urograms must be carefully evaluated at the time of simulation with the patient in the treatment position to assure the exact location of the kidney with respect to the edge of the radiation fields. If such care is taken to localize the kidneys properly, the risk of radiation-induced injury is essentially eliminated.

In patients with pure seminoma, megavoltage radiation doses in the range of 3000 rad in 4 weeks given in daily fractions of 150–200 rad, treating five sessions per week are adequate (*vide infra*). In areas of lymphographically positive nodes boosts of an additional 600 rad are given. In patients with extensive retroperitoneal seminoma (clinical Stage IIB) marginal recurrence is clearly higher than the incidence of local in-field recurrence.[4] Whole abdominal radiation therapy to doses of 2000 rad should be used at a rate of 150 rad/fraction (if tolerated) followed by field reduction such that at least 50% of the renal parenchyma is spared but bulk and nodal disease treated to 4000 rad. For patients with nonseminomatous testicular carcinoma who are treated with radiation therapy alone the dose should be in the range of 4500 rad in 5–6 weeks using 150–180 rad/fraction. Bulky retroperitoneal disease and extranodal disease from these tumors should be treated with initial chemotherapy often combined with adjuvant radiation therapy and/or surgery (*vide infra*).

Treatment of the mediastinum and supraclavicular regions should be carried out electively in patients with Clinical Stage II seminoma. Care to match these fields with the previously irradiated retroperitoneal portals should be done using appropriate gap, moving junction, and/or junctional wedge techniques commonly used now in the treatment of patients with testicular or lymphomatous malignancies. In addition the contralateral testis should be shielded with lead cups; these will usually reduce the gonadal dose due to scattered radiation to 1.0%–1.5% of that given to the retroperitoneum.

Symptomatically, retroperitoneal radiation therapy is quite well tolerated by the young men undergoing this treatment. They nearly always continue their work or education during treatment with very little interruption. Approximately half of the patients treated experience mild nausea, which is usually controlled with antiemetic medication. Very uncommonly is treatment interruption necessary for this side effect. Weekly hemograms are checked during such therapy, but at most only 20% require a treatment interruption for moderate, but never severe, leukopenia or thrombocytopenia. Acute radiation enteritis or colitis are uncommon in this dose range (3000–4500 rad) when given with conventional fractionation (150–200 rad), five sessions per week. If such symptoms occur, they are easily controlled with antispasmodic medication and subside shortly following the completion of treatment. Delayed or late gastrointestinal reactions such as radiation enteritis or bowel obstruction are rarely seen following such treatment, if they are not combined with a retroperitoneal lymph node resection.[7] All patients undergoing retroperitoneal radiation develop a reversible reduction in spermatogenesis secondary to the low level of scattered radiation (30–80 rad over 4–6 weeks). The resulting oligospermia persists for 12–18 months following radiation therapy, but sperm counts and fertility will in nearly all instances return to their preirradiated levels in 18–24 months.[20,21]

Radiation Therapy in the Management of Patients with Testicular Seminoma

Treatment Results and Recommendations

The exquisite sensitivity of the retroperitoneal lymph node metastases from pure seminoma following orchiectomy by external beam radiation therapy was reported three decades ago by Friedman.[22] A more recent analysis of the doses of megavoltage radiation therapy necessary to sterilize such metastatic deposits from pure seminoma confirm his original observations that 3000 rads given with the conventional fractionation (150–200 rad/day, 5 sessions/week) is virtually certain of sterilizing these metastases (Table I). Only one of 132 patients treated at the M. D. Anderson Hospital sustained an in-field local failure when a range of doses, varying with clinical settings, from 2000–4500 rad was used.[4] Local control of seminoma, like other tumors and normal tissue tolerance, depend on the time-dose relationships[23] rather than total dose alone. On review of our seminoma experience at this hospital since 1950 a para-aortic recurrence of seminoma (biopsy proven) occurred in one of 135 Stage I patients irradiated with megavoltage doses of 2300–3000 rad. However, the administration of this patients' radiation of 2300 rad had been uncommonly protracted over an interval of 5 weeks. The radiation sensitivity for the anaplastic seminoma, a pathologic variant of pure seminoma in which there is an unusually high incidence of mitoses per high power field, appears to be the same as in other types of seminoma.[5]

A review of the reported results of treating patients with clinical Stage I seminoma with external beam is shown in Table I. The combined 3-year disease-free survival of 603 patients reported from the five major treatment centers is 97% with a range of 94%–100%. Generally, these outstanding results were achieved without the mediastinal or left supraclavicular lymph nodal regions being radiated prophylactically. The patterns of failure were looked at specifically by the M. D. Anderson group in which they noted that only one of 59 patients treated without prophylactic radiation given supradiaphragmatically failed in this region.[4] The group from the Royal Marsden Hospital reported that in the minority of patients with seminoma in their series who did receive mediastinal radiation prophylactically there was a higher incidence of interrcurrent deaths due to myocardial infarctions than in the much larger group who did not receive radiation to this area.[6] Thus, although this was not a statistically significant difference and the median age of patients with seminoma is higher than that for patients with other testicular tumors, prophylactic treatment of the mediastinum in Clinical Stage I seminoma does not seem indicated.

The results of treating patients with Clinical Stage II pure seminoma by external beam radiation therapy is also shown in Table I. For the 164 patients reported the total 3-year disease-free survival was 85% with a range of 74%–93%. The treatment in nearly all instances included prophylactic radiation to the mediastinum and supraclavicular reigons usually to doses of 2000–3000 rad following the retroperitoneal treatment. Such treatment is to be highly recommended from the outstanding success rates. This is further supported by the limited data on patterns of failure from the M. D. Anderson Hospital, viz., in five patients with Stage II seminoma who did not receive mediastinal radiation therapy there were two incidences of failure in the supraclavicular nodes.[4] These results and the knowledge of the incidence of proven histologic involvement of the supraclavicular lymph nodes to be in the range of 15%–20% in patients with Clinical Stage

Table II.
Radiation Therapy in Nonseminomatous Testis Carcinoma

Institution	Clinical Stage I		Clinical Stage II	
	Number	% 3-year disease-free survival	Number	% 3-year disease-free survival
Royal Marsden Hospital[6,10]	102	85%	25[a]	76%
Walter Reed[29]	29	86%	11[a]	82%
Rotterdam Institute[8]	29	90%	35	45%
Stanford University[7]	14	79%	17[a]	58%
Total	174	86%	88	61%

[a] Patients with bulky nodal disease on lymphogram were generally excluded for treatment with radiation alone at these institutions and thus are not included in their reported series.

II testicular cancer by staging biopsy,[24,25] make this treatment essential in the management of patients with this stage disease. For patients with bulky retroperitoneal lymph node disease, modifications of the usual treatment techniques of the retroperitoneum are necessary. First, the whole abdominal cavity should be treated to doses in the range of 2000 rad to minimize the possibility of a marginal recurrence of these not infrequently extensively infiltrating tumors. Secondly, the boost dose to the bulk disease should be raised to levels of 4000 rads with careful shaping of the coned-down retroperitoneal fields to exclude 50%–70% of the renal parenchyma from receiving doses in excess of 2400 rad. Retroperitoneal exploration following radiation therapy of such bulk tumors should be considered when clinical regression of the tumor has not occurred or when, despite careful treatment planning, doses in the range of 4000 rad to the bulk disease cannot be given without the possibility of radiation compromise to more than 50% of the renal parenchyma.

Much less commonly, patients present with Clinical Stage III or IV seminoma, i.e., with clinical evidence of disease dissemination to the supradiaphragmatic lymphatics or to extralymphatic sites. The success rate in these patients treated with radiation therapy is less certain because of the small number of patients reported. This composite experience, however, suggests that over half of the patients treated with advanced stages can be cured with radiation therapy alone.[4,6,7] However, alkylating agent chemotherapy has been quite effective in disseminated seminoma and thus should be considered in the management of patients presenting with these advanced stages. Our present treatment policy with Stage III or IV patients is to treat with radiation therapy to all involved or potentially involved lymph nodal regions, usually supplemented with 1500-rad whole lung radiation, followed by a year of Cytoxan chemotherapy.

Treatment failures following radiation therapy for patients with seminoma occur as in other testicular tumors usually within the first 2 years of presentation.

Accordingly, patients are followed closely for 2 years by physical exam and chest x-rays (and serum markers if they were originally either positive or not done). Follow-up thereafter is done annually for 5 years. This initial close follow-up is felt advisable despite the high success rates of treatment with radiation therapy because should distant metastases develop, occasionally of nonseminomatous histology,[4] cure is still possible by further radiation therapy often combined with either surgery or chemotherapy.

Treatment Recommendations in Seminoma Patients with an Elevated HCG

The presence of a positive HCG by the relatively insensitive urinary bio-assay technique in five of 83 patients with seminoma treated at the Walter Reed Hospital 10–30 years ago predicted a lethal outcome in all five.[5] However, these five patients all presented with very advanced disease, and metastatic seminomatous masses did show the usual radiosensitivity to local therapy (Maier, personal communication). Subsequent to this experience the much more sensitive and specific (no interference with LH) radioimmunoassay to the beta subunit of HCG has been developed.[26] Prospective studies indicate quite conclusively that a small number of patients with pure seminoma do present with an elevated serum HCG by antibody assay to the beta subunit.[27,28] Javadpour and associates found an elevated HCG in 5% or three of 60 patients presenting with seminoma whose primary tumor was confirmed to be pure seminoma on review of serial histologic sectioning.[28] Immunoperoxidase staining of the primary tumor identified HCG within benign syncytiotrophoblastic giant cells associated with the seminoma.[28] In the one other patient in this series with an elevated HCG an element of choriocarcinoma was identified on serial histologic sectioning of the primary tumor. Any patient with an elevated AFP should be managed as having a nonseminomatous tumor as this appears to be diagnostic for the presence of embryonal carcinoma or yolk-sac tumor.[14,28]

Our experinece and that reported by others,[19,27] all with follow-up limited to less than 5 years, has been that patients with pure seminoma and an elevated HCG have metastatic masses with the usual excellent radiosensitivity and are all in maintained complete remission following treatment. In the last 5 years we have irradiated four patients (Stage I-2, Stage IIB-1, Stage IV-1) with pure seminoma (on review of histologic step-sections) and an elevated serum HCG. All are in complete remission, both clinically and serologically. The Stage IIB patient who had a 9 × 5 × 5 right retroperitoneal mass obstructing completely the right ureter and common iliac vein was treated with 2000 rad to the whole abdomen, 3600 rad to the retroperitoneal lymph nodes, and a boost to the original bulky disease to 4000 rad. 2600 rad of elective irradiation was given to the mediastinum and supraclavicular region. At the completion of the retroperitoneal irradiation his serum HCG was negative, and repeat ultrasound showed clearance of the obstructing mass. Two months later a retroperitoneal exploration revealed no mass, and all sectioned tissue was fibrotic and free of tumor. He remains free of disease now $3\frac{1}{2}$ years following diagnosis. The Stage IV patient who had even more massive retroperitoneal disease and a 5 cm pulmonary mass (cytologically seminoma on skinny-needle biopsy) is in complete clinical and serologic remission 1 year following similar treatment plus lung irradiation and Cytoxan chemotherapy.

Thus, our present treatment strategy is similar to that recommended by Whitmore[14] for patients with pure seminoma and an elevated serum HCG. If step-sectioning of the primary tumor fails to demonstrate any nonseminomatous tumor elements, the treatment is by radiation therapy employing the same fields and doses as is usual for the patients' clinical stage. If the HCG remains elevated, then additional treatment by surgery and/or chemotherapy is essential.

Management of Patients with Nonseminomatous Testicular Carcinoma

Results of Radiation Therapy

In comparing the results of surgery and radiation therapy in the treatment of the retroperitoneal lymph nodes in patients with nonseminomatous testicular cancer, critical attention must be given to the method of staging the presence or absence of metastases in these lymph nodes. Clinical staging (primarily lymphangiographic) is 70%–80% accurate when compared to surgical or pathologic staging on the basis of radical retroperitoneal node dissection.[15–18] Radiation series including information of preirradiation serum HCG and AFP are not yet available. Patients who are lymphangiographically evaluated as Stage I include a subgroup of approximately 20% who have microscopic metastases to one or more retroperitoneal lymph nodes. Therefore, if direct comparison of the results of retroperitoneal treatment techniques (surgery, radiation or a combination of both) is to be attempted, then the groups must be matched for initial clinical stage. Unfortunately, all surgical series, with the exception of that recently reported from M. D. Anderson Hospital,[11] do not report their results of retroperitoneal node dissection by initial clinical stage. Thus, most surgical series report only by pathologic stage and hence the extent of disease at each stage is less in the surgical series than in the clinical staging reported for treatment with radiation therapy alone.

The results of radiation therapy alone for the treatment of the retroperitoneal lymph nodes for patients with Clinical Stage I nonseminomatous testicular cancer is shown in Table II. 174 patients reported from these four institutions document the 3-year disease-free survival following radiation therapy alone is 86% with a range of 79%–90%.[6–8,10,29] The survival results by histologic subtype for Stage I patients is reported in the Royal Marsden Hospital series and appears better for patients with teratocarcinoma, 31 or 97% of 32, than for those with embryonal carcinoma, 24 or 77% of 31.[6] A similar result is seen in the Rotterdam series,[8] although from this report only the combined Stage I and II patients are compared by histologic subtype, i.e., from the data available a 75% survival is reported in 44 patients with teratocarcinoma (Dixon and Moore, Group III) compared to 53% of 32 patients with embryonal carcinoma (Dixon and Moore, Group IV). These results are comparable to those reported by surgery alone for patients with pathologically Stage I testicular carcinoma with such series reporting usually a 3-year disease-free survival ranging from 80% to 100%.[1,11,30–34] When reported in these surgical series, a similar trend in survival advantage was seen for patients with teratocarcinoma compared to those with embryonal carcinoma.

A comparison of the patterns of failure for patients presenting with Clinical Stage I disease treated by radiation, surgery or a combination of both the retroperitoneal lymph nodes is shown in Table III. The incidence of retroperitoneal failure is low by either surgery or radiation therapy—5% or less. The incidence for subsequent development of distant metastases for patients with Clinical Stage I disease is likewise found to be comparable—approximately 10%—although this may be able to be reduced by the use of preoperative radiation therapy (2500–3000 rad), but seemingly not so by use of postoperative radiation. The role of mediastinal and supraclavicular prophylactic radiation in these Stage I patients with a high cure (3-year disease-free survival) rate and the low incidence of distant metastases is uncertain. Radiation to the level of 4000 rad prophylactically to these regions was generally given to the patients in Clinical Stage I reported in Tables II and III, except for the group treated by surgery alone. In view of the proven efficacy of multidrug chemotherapy which requires a substantial bone marrow reserve, the practice of administering prophylactic supradiaphragmatic radiation in clinical Stage I to the patients treated with radiation therapy for nonseminomatous testicular tumors should be critically reevaluated and likely, as in seminoma, discontinued.

The results of radiation therapy alone in the treatment of 88 patients with clinical Stage II disease showed a 3-year disease-free survival of 61% with a range of 45%–82% (Table II). Patients selected for this treatment at the four radiation centers reporting their results were biased towards those patients having relatively minimal metastatic retroperitoneal disease by lymphangiogram (Stage IIA). However, this was not the case with the group reported from Rotterdam where radiation therapy alone was used in patients with bulky retroperitoneal disease (Stage IIB) without combining it with a planned surgical resection (van der Werf-Messing, personal communication). Thus, cure rates for patients with minimally positive lymphangiograms, usually with involvement of nodes less than 2 cm in greatest diameter,[12] range from 58% to 82%. These results, allowing for differences in staging techniques, compare favorably with the similar survival results of 60%–86% reported for patients with resectable pathologic Stage II disease following lymphadenectomy alone[1,30–33,36] despite the fact that some selection has occurred in the surgical series. Specifically, the patients reported in these series often do not include those that have disease above the level of the renal arteries and whose disease was found to be "unresectable" at exploration.

Table III.

Patterns of Failure in Nonseminomatous Testis Carcinoma

Institution	Treatment	Retroperitoneal recurrence	Distant metastasis
Clinical Stage I:			
Royal Marsden Hospital[12]	RT alone	4/85 — 5%	9/85 — 11%
M. D. Anderson Hospital[11]	Surgery alone	2.89 — 2%	9/89 — 10%
M. D. Anderson Hospital[11]	Surg. + postop RT	1/17 — 6%	3/17 — 18%
M. D. Anderson Hospital[11] + Walter Reed[29,35]	Preop RT + Surgery	0/35 — 0%	1/35 — 3%
Clinical Stage IIA:			
Royal Marsden Hospital	RT alone	1/14 — 7%	3/14 – 21%
M. D. Anderson Hospital	Surgery alone	4/6 — 67%	2/6 — 33%
M. D. Anderson Hospital	Surg. + postop RT	2/12 — 17%	6/12 — 50%
M. D. Anderson Hospital + Walter Reed	Preop RT + Surgery[a]	0/39 — 0%	8/39 — 20%
Clinical Stage IIB:			
Royal Marsden Hospital	RT alone	9/13 — 69%	10/15 — 67%
M. D. Anderson Hospital	Preop RT + Surgery[b]	1/7 — 14%	4/7 — 57%

[a] About one-half of these patients received additional RT postoperatively.
[b] Most patients also received postoperative RT.

Combining postoperative radiation therapy with surgical resection appears from results of retrospective studies not to be superior to treatment either by surgery or radiation therapy alone.[1,7,11,37,38] In the Stage II category patients with teratocarcinoma seem to have better survival than those with embryonal carcinoma whether they are treated by radiation alone[6] or by retroperitoneal dissection with or without adjuvant radiation therapy or chemotherapy.[1,31,32]

The patterns of failure for patients with Clinical Stage IIA disease with regional therapy by radiation, surgery, or a combination of the two are outlined in Table III. Radiotherapy alone with well-tolerated doses of 4500 rad in 5–6 weeks yielded

Table IV.

Prognostic Value of Preoperative Radiation.

Clinical Stage II Nonseminomatous Testis Carcinoma

Lymph node Histology	Incidence of distant metastases		
	M. D. Anderson[9]	Walter Reed[23,29]	Total
Negative	1/13	0/10	1/23 — 4%
Positive	3/5	4/11	7/16 — 44%

excellent local control (93%). Only one patient (with embryonal carcinoma) failed in the retroperitoneal nodes of 14 treated.[12] The accuracy (true positive rate) of lymphangiography in Stage IIA patients is 90%.[11,17] Thus, radiation therapy alone in doses of 4500 rad sterilized all retroperitoneal nodal disease in 11 of 12 or about 90% of these patients. The data for local control by surgery alone in clinical Stage IIA patients is difficult to find in the literature because very few patients are treated by surgery alone and many surgical series do not report their local failure rates. Thus, the small number of patients reported in Table III may be too few to allow meaningful evaluation. The incidence of local failure is likely to be reduced by postoperative radiation therapy as shown from an 83% local success rate with this combined approach. However, 50% of these patients developed disseminated disease.[11] The incidence of distant metastases in patients treated with radiation therapy alone or with preoperative radiation therapy and retroperitoneal node dissection was approximately 20%. This is substantially lower than can be inferred from previously reported survival figures of 50%–60% for pathologic Stage II patients treated with surgery and postoperative radiation therapy.[7,37,38] In addition preoperative radiation therapy (2500–3000 rad) and surgical resection seems to offer a clear superiority in local control. Specifically, there were no local recurrences in the 39 patients so treated by the group at the M. D. Anderson Hospital and the Walter Reed Hospital (Table III). While these good results with regard to local control rate and impressively low incidence of distant metastases may be unique to these two institutions and may reflect some patient selection, this experience more likely suggests that surgical dissection of active disease in the para-aortic lymph nodes may lead to dissemination which can be prevented by preoperative radiation therapy.

Further, preoperative radiation therapy in the range of 2500–3000 rad primarily in patients with clinical Stage IIA disease yields a significant incidence of pathologic downstaging in the surgically resected lymph nodes. In patients with clinical Stage IIA disease at the M. D. Anderson Hospital, 89% or 16 of 18 patients without preoperative radiation therapy had positive lymph nodes in their resected specimens while only 28% or 5 of 18 patients treated with 2500–3000 rad preoperatively had histological evidence of metastases in the resected lymph nodes.[11] In the Walter Reed series only 52% or 11 of the 21 clinical Stage II patinets treated had histologically positive nodes following 2500 rads of preoperative radiation therapy.[29,35] These data indicate that 2500–3000 rad can cause immediate marked regression of the metastases in the retroperitoneal lymph nodes and is able to render them free of histologically detectable tumor cells in the majority of instances. This, in addition to the 93% local control rate in the retroperitoneal nodes of patients with clinical Stage IIA disease treated with 4500 rad[12] is documentation of the radiation sensitivity of nonseminomatous testicular tumors. Further, pathologic downstaging to N_0 following preoperative radiation therapy is likely a favorable prognostic sign in patients with nonseminomatous testicular carcinoma as it is in bladder carcinoma.[39,40] Table IV shows a review of the combined experience from the M. D. Anderson and Walter Reed Hospitals on the prognostic value of downstaging by preoperative irradiation. Only one or 4% of 23 patients found to be pathologically downstaged to N_0 following radiation therapy subsequently developed distant metastasis compared to the significantly higher rate of subsequent distant failure in patients who did not have histologic irradiation of their tumor with those doses of preoperative radiation therapy (i.e., in 44% or 7 of 16 patients).[11,29,35] Thus, the presences or absence of pathologic downstaging following preoperative radiation therapy would seem to be a good method to select patients for consideration of adjuvant chemotherapy, as has been used in bladder cancer.[41,42]

The available published data on patterns of failure of patients with clinical Stage IIB nonseminomatous testicular cancer indicate that treatment results are unfavorable in this group if they are treated with nonsystemic therapy (Table III). Radiation therapy alone for this bulk disease is clearly inferior to radiation followed by surgical resection. Approximately two-thirds of the patients in this group will develop metastases regardless of local therapy, and thus this advanced group of patients should be candidates for early multidrug adjuvant chemotherapy because their risk of developing distant metastases is so high.

Comparison of the Common Sequellae of Treatment by Surgery, Radiation Therapy, or Chemotherapy

The common, and the unlikely, sequellae of lymph node dissection, external beam irradiation, the multidrug chemotherapy must be critically analyzed and appreciated prior to recommendation of these treatment modalities. Table V outlines the major toxicities known to be associated with each modality.

Retroperitoneal node dissection usually causes permanent infertility from nonejaculatory orgasm because of surgical damage to the autonomic nerves in the retroperitoneum.[19,21,31,34] This complication, however, is not reported following staging laparotomy for Hodgkin's disease in which only a selected sampling of the retroperitoneal lymph nodes is carried out.[13] Uncommonly erectile impotence can also occur due to the surgical interruption of autonomic nerves below the aortic and caval bifurcations. Neither surgery nor anesthesia compromise the bone marrow reserve. However, the unusually low incidence of distant metastases (20%) reported for patients with Clinical Stage II disease who were treated by preoperative radiation therapy and retroperitoneal lymph node dissection raises the distinct possibility that surgical resection of active disease in the lymph nodes can lead to tumor cell dissemination.

External beam radiation, even in the presence of careful shielding, results in the radiation of the contralateral testis to 1% to 1.5% of the prescribed dose by internally scattered photons. Such unavoidable irradiation (usually 45–80 rad over 4–6 weeks) causes a temporary marked reduction in spermatogenesis and fertility.[20,21] However, complete recovery of the resulting oligospermia with return to pretreatment levels of the patient's sperm count and fertility consistently occur by 18 months following radiation.[20,21] Some residual genetic damage in

Table V.

Common Sequella of Treatment in Patients with Testicular Carcinoma

| Treatment | Sequellae | |
	Fertility	Bone marrow reserve
Surgery		
Staging lymph node sampling	No compromise	No compromise
Radical lymph node dissection	Permanent loss (nonejaculatory orgasm; impotence, rare)	No compromise
Irradiation		
Retroperitoneal fields only (4500 rad)	Temporary loss (oligospermia; 12–18 months)	No significant compromise
Multiple fields (including mediastinal and supra-clavicular fields)	Temporary loss (oligospermia; 12–18 months)	Likely moderate compromise
Chemotherapy		
Single agent	Effect uncertain	Likely moderate compromise
Multiple agents	Permanent loss (aspermia)	Severe compromise

the fertile mature gamete 2 years following treatment may remain, and patients should be so advised, although clinical evidence for it in this setting has not been reported. Prior irradiation only to retroperitoneal fields causes some reduction in bone marrow reserve,[43] but this level of damage does not preclude effective combination chemotherapy, although prior chemotherapy has.[10,44] However, if irradiation is to both retroperitoneal and supradiaphragmatic ports, then bone marrow tolerance for the effective multidrug chemotherapy regimens is likely to be significantly reduced, as has been reported by some centers in combining MOPP chemotherapy and total nodal radiation in patients with Hodgkin's disease.[45]

Multidrug chemotherapy has in the treatment of boys and young men with lymphoma resulted in irreversible aspermia.[46,4,7] This effect is not surprising because, unlike irradiation, the remaining gonad cannot be shielded from 98% of the given dose.

The combination of retroperitoneal node dissection with full-dose radiation (usually 4500 rad by a "sandwich" technique) has been reported to result in a significant (~15%) incidence of late intestinal complications.[7] This incidence is a rare complication in the treatment of Hodgkin's disease where lymph node sampling is combined with these doses of irradiation.[13] Thus, when retroperitonea' treatment by both surgery and radiation therapy is planned, reduction in the intensity of one or both of these modalities should be encouraged. However, it is noteworthy that the combination of retroperitoneal node dissection and multidrug chemotherapy is not likely to cause any increase in morbidity over that which can be expected from their individual toxicities. In fact, as both chemotherapy and retroperitoneal node dissection cause infertility (but for different reasons), the probability of this sequellae is unlikely to be increased by combining the two modalities.

The possibility of causing, with a very low probability, a subsequent hematologic or other maliganacy from the use of known oncogenic agents such as radiation and chemotherapy in these young men is difficult to evaluate. However, the recent review of the significant incidence of leukemia after treatment with alkylating agent chemotherapy, but not after radiation therapy alone, in women with ovarian carcinoma makes adjuvant treatment with these chemotherapeutic agents at least a worrisome consideration at this point.[48]

Recommendations for Treatment

Based on the analysis of the above data in patients with nonseminomatous testicular cancer on therapeutic efficacy for relapse-free survival, for patterns of failure, and for treatment-related toxicities, the following treatment recommendations are made:

1. *Patients with clinical Stage I disease:* radiation therapy to the para-aortic and ipsilateral iliac and inguinal lymph nodes to doses of 4500 rad in 5–6 weeks. This approach gives cure rates equal to surgery and would allow the preservation of potency, ejaculation, and fertility in the majority of patients treated. However, prior to recommending radiation therapy as the effective treatment that should preserve fertility, it is important to check that the patient has an adequate sperm profile since frequently patients with testicular tumors have a low fertility status.[49] Following radiation serum markers and chest films should be followed closely for at least 2 years to detect disease activation early should it develop. If either the serum HCG or AFP is elevated prior to radiation and either does not become normal within 1 month following completion of the radiation therapy, then further treatment with either chemotherapy or surgery is indicated. In the 10%–15% of patients (likely somewhat less in those with teratocarcinoma and more in those with embryonal carcinoma) who subsequently develop evidence of distant metastases, multidrug chemotherapy will be possible provided that the radiation therapy has been only to the lymph nodal regions below the diaphragm.

2. *Patients with clinical Stage IIA disease:* preoperative radiation therapy to the para-aortic and ipsilateral iliac and inguinal lymph nodes to doses of 2500–3000 rad followed by lymphadenectomy seems the best available approach. This achieves excellent local control of the retroperitoneal lymph node disease (Table III) and further allows the presence or absence of pathologic downstaging to assist in the selection for adjuvant chemotherapy only those patients who are

at particularly high risk of developing distant metastases. Because of the efficacy of adjuvant preoperative radiation therapy, a strong consideration should be given to reducing the extent of the surgical resection to allow preservation of ejaculatory orgasm and thus fertility in this group of young men who have high likelihood of cure. However, the extent of the possible reduction in the usual surgical dissection will likely have to be cautiously individualized because the site of possible retroperitoneal nodal metastasis is variable and unpredictable.[19] Further, additional consideration for the routine use of staging supraclavicular lymph node biopsy for the detection of occult supradiaphragmatic metastases seem warranted in these patients. Both Donohue[25] and Buck[24] have documented the incidence of occult supraclavicular lymph nodal metastases to be between 15% and 20% in these patients. In those patients with surgically proven dissemination to the supraclavicular lymph nodes initiation of multidrug chemotherapy promptly would seem indicated which should subsequently be combined with either surgery or radiation therapy for possible residual retroperitoneal disease;

3. *Patients presenting with clinical Stage IIB, III, or IV disease:* the high incidence of development of systemic metastases warrants initiation of treatment by multidrug chemotherapy. Following a course of chemotherapy that is likely to achieve a complete response[44,50] and whose duration would be until maximum response was likely to have been achieved, surgery and/or radiation therapy should be used as felt necessary for control of possible residual disease. The best method of combining local therapies after the initial multidrug chemotherapy in patients with clinical Stage IIB, III, and IV disease would be an excellent topic for a prospective multi-institutional clinical trial if all physicians caring for these patients agree on such a study;

4. Clearly the probabilities of the "correctness" of the above clinical stages can be improved by the knowledge of and experience with serum markers—HCG and AFP—taken before and after orchiectomy. In addition, in all stages where a serum marker was initially positive the response to a therapy can be well followed for both the achievement of a complete response and the possible early detection of a recurrence.

Finally, treatment must in all instances be individualized with the patient appraised of the rationale, potential risks, and benefits of all alternative therapies such that he can share in the decision-making process as this seems both ethical and important to the patients' physical and psychological outlook.[51,52]

Possible Future Developments in Radiation Technique

Optimizing technique to minimize damage to normal tissue in radiation therapy, as has been well appreciated for decades in surgery, can favorably influence patient tolerance and recovery. Further improvements in our present techniques to irradiate the retroperitoneal lymph nodes, which could lower the dose to the lumbar and pelvic bone marrow, may come from treatment plans with multiple contoured fields and/or by the use of charged particle beam irradiation.

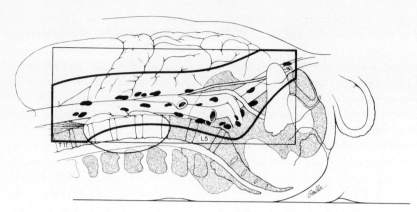

FIGURE 2. Contoured lateral radiation treatment field for patients with clinical Stage I or IIA testicular cancer but without epididymal involvement or prior inguinal surgery.

Reduced irradiation of bone marrow (in both dose and volume) will improve patient tolerance for subsequent combination chemotherapy, should this be necessary. Such chemotherapy is effective in irradicating metastases, but this treatment has severe, occasionally life-threatening, hematologic toxicity.[44,50]

The depth-dose characteristics and the relatively sharp beam edge of high-energy (10–25 MV) linear accelerators allow treatment by individually shaped lateral fields for a portion of the retroperitoneal irradiation (Fig. 2). These fields spare more of the axial bone marrow that is posterior to the retroperitoneal nodes and also give less irradiation to the abdominal viscera. However, because of the well-known level of renal radiation tolerance (2400–2800 rad), only 1500 rad of the total dose should be administered by these portals. We have found this approach well tolerated in patients with Stage IIA disease irradiated preoperatively to 3000 rad followed in 3–4 weeks by lymphadenectomy.

Further improvements in radiation dose distribution to spare the lumbar and pelvic bone marrow may come from the use of charged particle beam irradiation. Charged particles all have the advantage of a finite distance of penetration in tissue depending on their initial energy. Because of this unique depth dose characteristic very favorable dose distributions can, or potentially could, be achieved in treating the retroperitoneal lymph nodal region. These charged particles include: 1) electrons, usually produced from betatrons or linear accelerators that are available in most major treatment centers, and 2) protons, pions, and heavy ions (helium, carbon, and nitrogen), which are being developed and evaluated at only a few centers in the world. Theoretical treatment plans have been designed for proton, pion, and heavy particle beams that will be able to treat the retroperitoneum with the bone marrow in the lumbar spine receiving only 10%–20% of the dose administered to the tumor volume.[53] However, the clinical achievement of such schemes is likely some years away.

The use of electrons for retroperitoneal irradiation with improved sparing of the lumbar spine and pelvic bone marrow is a method that is now potentially available. However, because of the limited penetration (3–5 cm) of high energy (12–18 MeV) electrons, this irradiation must be delivered *intra*operatively directly to the retroperitoneal region. Using a 12- or 15-MeV electron beam, a homogeneous single dose to the retroperitoneal nodes of 1000 rad would give only 300–400 rad to the more posteriorly located bone marrow of the lumbar spine and pelvis. Such single shot *intra*operative electron beam therapy has been given effectively and safely to patients with a variety of abdominal and pelvic tumors and to the retroperitoneal lymph nodes in Japan,[54,55] at Howard University, and at our institution (32 patients), but not as yet to patients with nodal metastases from testicular carcinoma. However, such an *intra*operative approach would combine the attractive advantages 1) of a favorable dose distribution that would avoid irradiating the intestine and reduce substantially the dose to the lumbar and pelvic bone marrow, and 2) if such irradiation were given immediately prior to the surgical lymph node dissection, then this could minimize the chance of intraoperative seeding of tumor cells, but not alter the accuracy of the pathologic staging.

References

1. Whitmore, W. F., Jr.: Germinal tumors of the testis. *Proceedings of the 6th National Cancer Conference*. Philadelphia: J. B. Lippincott Co., 1970.

2. Prout, G. R., Jr.: Germinal tumors of the testis. *Cancer Medicine* Holland, James F. and Frei, Emil III (Eds.). Philadelphia: Lee and Febiger, 1973, pp. 1696–1708.

3. Dixon, F. J., and Moore, R. A.: Tumors of the male sex organs. *Atlas of Tumor Pathology*, Section VIII, FAS 31b and 32. Washington, D. C.: Armed Forces Institute of Pathology, 1952.

4. Doornbos, J. F., Hussey, D. H., and Johnson, D. E.: Radiotherapy for pure seminoma of the testis. *Radiology* **116**:401–404, 1975.

5. Maier, J. G., and Sulak, M. H.: Radiation therapy in malignant testis tumors, Part I, Seminoma. *Cancer* **32**:1212–1216, 1973.

6. Peckham, M. J., and McElwain, T. J.: Radiotherapy of testicular tumors. *Proc R Soc Med* **67**:300–303, 1974.

7. Earle, J. D., Bagshaw, M. A., and Kaplan, H. S.: Supervoltage radiation therapy of testicular tumors. *Am J Roentgenol* **117**:653–661, 1973.

8. van der Werf-Messing, B.: Radiotherapeutic treatment of testicular tumors. *Int J Radiat Oncol* **1**:235–248, 1976.

9. Maier, J. G., and Lee, S. N.: Radiation therapy for nonseminomatous germ cell testicular cancer in adults. *Urol Clin North Am* **4**:477–493, 1977.

10. Peckham, M. J.: An appraisal of the role of radiation therapy in the management of nonseminomatous germ cell tumors of the testis in the era of effective chemotherapy. *Cancer Treat Rev*: in press, 1979.

11. Hussey, D. H., Luk, K. H., and Johnson, D. E.: The role of radiation therapy in the treatment of germinal cell tumors of the testis other than pure seminoma. *Radiology* **123**:175–180, 1977.

12. Tyrrell, C. J., and Peckham, M. J.: The response of lymph node metastases of testicular teratoma to radiation therapy. *Br J Urol* **48**:363–370, 1976.

13. Kaplan, H. S.: *Hodgkin's Disease*. Cambridge, Mass.: Harvard University Press, 1972.

14. Barzell, W. E., and Whitmore, W. F., Jr.: Clinical significance of biological markers in non-seminomatous germinal testis tumors: Memorial Hospital experience. *Seminars in Oncology*. In press, 1979.

15. Wallace, S., and Jing, B. S.: Lymphangiography: diagnosis of lymph node metastases from testicular malignancies. *J Am Med Assoc* **213**:94–97, 1970.

16. Maier, J. G., and Schamber, D. T.: The role of lymphangiography in the diagnosis and treatment of malignant testicular tumors. *Am J Roentgenol* **114**:482–491, 1972.

17. Ray, B., Hajdu, S. I., and Whitmore, W. F., Jr.: Distribution of retroperitoneal lymph node metastases in testicular germinal tumors. *Cancer* **32**:340–348, 1974.

18. Safer, M. L., Green, J. P., Crews, Q. E., Jr., and Hill, D. R.: Lymphangiographic accuracy in staging of testicular tumors. *Cancer* **35**:1603–1605, 1975.

19. Whitmore, W. F., Jr.: Surgical treatment of adult germinal testis tumors. *Seminars in Oncologyl*. In press, 1979.

20. Smithers, D. W., Wallace, D. M., and Austin, D. E.: Fertility after unilateral orchiectomy and radiotherapy for patients with malignant tumours of the testis. *Br Med J* **4**:77–79, 1973.

21. Orecklin, J. R., Kaufman, J. J., and Thompson, R. W.: Fertility in patients treated for malignant testicular tumors. *J Urol* **109**:293–295, 1973.

22. Friedman, M.: Tumors of the testis and their treatment. *Clinical Therapeutic Radiology*. Portmann, U. V. (Ed.). New York: Nelson Thomas and Sons, 1950.

23. Ellis, F.: Nominal standard dose and the ret. *Br J Rad* **44**:101–108, 1971.

24. Buck, A. S., Schramber, C. T., Maier, J. G., and Lewis, E. L.: Supraclavicular node biopsy and malignant testicular tumors. *J Urol* **107**:619–621, 1972.

25. Donohue, R. E., Pfister, R. R., Weigel, J. W., and Stonington, O. G.: Supraclavicular node biopsy in testicular tumors. *J Urol* **9**:546–548, 1977.

26. Vaitukaitis, J. L., Braunstein, G. D. and Ross, G. T.: The radio-immunoassay which specifically measures human chorionic gonadotrophin in the presence of human luteinizing hormone. *Am J Obstet Gynecol* **113**:751–758, 1972.

27. Lang, P. H. and Fraley, E. E.: Serum alpha-fetoprotein and human chorionic gonadotrophin in the treatment of patients with testicular tumors. *Urol Clin North Am* **4**:393–406, 1977.

28. Javadpour, N., McIntire, K. R., Waldmann, T. A., and Bergman, S. M.: Role of alpha-fetoprotein and human chorionic gonadotrophin in seminoma. *J Urol* **120**:687–690, 1978.

29. Maier, J. G., and Mittemeyer, B. T.: Carcinoma of the testis. *Cancer* **39**:981–986, 1977.

30. Skinner, D. G., and Leadbetter, W. F.: The surgical management of testis tumors. *J Urol* **106**:84–93, 1971.

31. Walsh, P. C. Kaufman, J. J., Coulson, W. F., and Goodwin, W. E.: Retroperitoneal lymphadenectomy for testicular tumors. *J Am Med Assoc* **217**:309–312, 1971.

32. Staubitz, W. J., Earley, K. S., Magoss, I. V., and Murphy, J. T.: Surgical treatment of nonseminomatous testis tumors. *Cancer* **32**:1206–1214, 1973.

33. Skinner, D. G.: Nonseminomatous testis tumors. *J Urol* **115**:65–70, 1976.

34. Donohue, J. P.: Retroperitoneal lymphadenectomy: The anterior approach including bilateral super-renal dissection. *Urol Clin North Am* **4**:509–522, 1977.

35. Klein, K. A., and Maier, J. G.: Positive nodes and treatment failures in testicular carcinomas. *Int J Radiat Oncol* **2**:1229–1231, 1977.

36. Donohue, J. P., Einhorn, L. H., and Perez, J. M.: Improved management of nonseminomatous testis tumor. *Cancer* **42**:2903–2908, 1978.

37. Nicholson, T. C., Walsh, P. E., and Rotner, M. B.: Lymphadenectomy combined with preoperative and postoperative cobalt 60 teletherapy in the management of embryonal carcinoma and teratocarcinoma of the testis. *J Urol* **112**:109–111, 1974.

38. Maier, J. G., and Sulak, M. H.: Radiation therapy in malignant testis tumors, Part II: Carcinoma. *Cancer* **32**:1217–1225, 1973.

39. Prout, G. R., Jr.: The surgical management of bladder carcinoma. *Urol Clin North Am* **3**:149–175, 1976.

40. Wallace, D. N., and Bloom, H. J. G.: The management of deeply infiltrating bladder carcinoma: Control trial of radical radiotherapy vs preoperative radiation therapy and radical cystectomy. *Br J Urol* **48**:587–594, 1976.

41. Cummings, K. B., Shipley, W. U., Einstein, A. B., and Cutler, S. J.: Current concepts in the management of patients with deeply invasive bladder carcinoma. *Seminars in Oncology.* In press, 1979.

42. Chan, R. C., and Johnson, D. E.: The role of preoperative irradiation in patients selection for chemotherapy trials in bladder cancer, presented at the Conference on Combined Modalities: Chemotherapy/Radiation Therapy, November 15–18, 1978. Hilton Head, South Carolina p. 60.

43. Hellman, S., and Fink, M. E.: Granulocyte reserve following radiation therapy as studied by the response to a bacterial endotoxin. *Blood* **25**:310–324, 1975.

44. Cheng, E., Cvitkovic, E., Wittes, R. E., and Golby, R. B.: Germ cell tumors (II) VABII in metastatic testicular cancer. *Cancer* **42**:2162–2168, 1978.

45. Prosnitz, L. R., Farber, L. R., Fischer, J. J., Bertino, J. R., and Fischer, D. B.: Long-term remissions with combined modality for advanced Hodgkin's disease. *Cancer* **37**:2826–2833, 1976.

46. Roeser, H. P., Stocks, A. E., and Smith, A. J.: Testicular damage due to cytotoxic drugs and recovery after cessation of therapy. *Aust NZ J Med* **3**:250–254, 1977.

47. Jones, P. H. M., Han, I. M., Marsden, H. B., Lendon, M. and Shalet, J. H.: Testicular biopsy and testicular function following therapy for acute lymphoblastic leukemia. *Proc Am Soc Clin Oncol* **19**:365, 1978.

48. Reimer, R. R., Hoover, R., Fraumeni, J. F., Jr., and Young, R. C.: Acute leukemia after alkylating-agent therapy of ovarian cancer. *N Engl J Med* **297**:177–181, 1977.

49. Skinner, D. G.: Advances in the management of non-seminomatous germinal tumors of the testis. *Br J Urol* **49**:553–560, 1977.

50. Einhorn, L. H. and Dononue, J. P.: Improved chemotherapy and disseminated testicular cancer. *J Urol* **117**:65–69, 1977.

51. Bok, S.: *Lying: Moral Choice in Public and Private Life.* New York: Pantheon Books, Inc., 1978.

52. Fiore, N.: Fighting cancer—one patient's perspective. *N. Engl J Med* **300**:284–289, 1979.

53. Bagshaw, M. A.: Particle radiation therapy: Thresholds of a new age for treatment of cancer with ionizing radiation. *N Engl J Med:* In press, 1979.

54. Abe, M., Takahashi, M., Yabumuto, E., *et al.*: Techniques, indications, and results of intraoperative electron beam radiotherapy of advanced cancers. *Ther Radiol* **116**:693–698, 1975.

55. Iwasaki, Y., Ohto, M., Todoroki, T., *et al.*: The treatment of carcinoma of the biliary system. *Surg Gynecol Obstet* **144**:219–224, 1977.

4

Tumor Markers in Testicular Tumor: Current Status and Future Prospects

Paul H. Lange, M.D.

Veterans Administration Medical Center; Department of Urologic Surgery, University of Minnesota Health Sciences Center, Minneapolis, Minnesota; Junior Faculty Fellow, American Cancer Society

K. Robert McIntire, M.D.

Diagnosis Branch, Division of Cancer Biology and Diagnosis, National Cancer Institute, National Institutes of Health, Bethesda, Maryland

Thomas A. Waldmann, M.D.

Metabolism Branch, Division of Cancer Biology and Diagnosis, National Cancer Institute, National Institutes of Health, Bethesda, Maryland

IT IS NOW WELL ESTABLISHED that the sensitive radioimmunoassays for alpha-fetoprotein (AFP) and human chorionic gonadotropin (hCG) have significantly altered the diagnosis and management of germ cell testicular tumors especially nonseminomatous germ cell testicular tumors (NSGCT).[1-3] However, recognition of their importance does not automatically enable the physician to use these tumor markers successfully. Accordingly, one purpose of this article is to review the clinical aspects of AFP/hCG determinations in testicular tumor, especially those little-appreciated nuances that often become very important in the clinical setting.

It is probably accurate to say that AFP and hCG, when measured together, are the best serum tumor markers in human oncology today. Despite this accolade, it is becoming apparent that work on markers in testicular tumor is only beginning. Thus the second purpose of this report is to acquaint the reader with some of this new work and to speculate about the future directions of this expanding field.

The data and opinions expressed here are based on our experience with these markers over the last 5 years in approximately 300 testicular tumor patients, of whom 200 had serial determinations, usually monthly. A majority of these marker determinations were made using the radioimmunoassays of the National Cancer Institute,[4,5] although a significant number in recent years were made using our own AFP assay[6] and an hCG assay of a commercial laboratory, both of which had been previously determined by us to be reliable clinically.

For the purpose of this article, stages of testicular tumor will be designated as follows: Stage I—tumor limited to the testis, epididymis, or spermatic cord; Stage II—tumor metastatic to the retroperitoneum only; and Stage III—metastatic disease extending beyond the retroperitoneum.

Background of AFP and hCG

Since there have been numerous excellent reviews relating fundamental facts about these two markers,[7,8] only those aspects pertinent to this article will be repeated. Alpha-fetoprotein is a glycoprotein of approximately 70,000 molecular weight which is produced by the fetal yolk sac, liver, and gastrointestinal tract of many species. In the human fetus, AFP is a major serum protein often reaching levels of 3 mg/ml at about the twelfth week of gestation and then diminishing so that after 1 year of age it is undetectable by the older and less sensitive methods of measurement and by new radioimmunoassays is usually less than 16 ng/ml. Its function is unknown, although it probably acts as an albuminlike serum protein in the fetus. It has been suggested that AFP also serves an immunoregulatory purpose, but the evidence for this is still not conclusive.[9]

In 1963, AFP was found in the sera of animals with chemically induced hepatomas, and soon thereafter it was detected in the sera of many patients with hepatomas and occasionally in patients with testicular teratocarcinoma. Using radioimmunoassays which are sensitive to as little as 1–5 ng/ml of AFP, this marker was found to be present in 70% of patients with hepatoma and also in about 70% of patients with teratocarcinoma or embryonal cell carcinoma. However, with increased sensitivity came decreased specificity, and in addition to testicular tumor and hepatomas, AFP by radioimmunoassay was found in patients with ataxia telangiectasia; in hereditary tyrosinemia; in some patients with pancreatic, biliary, and other gastrointestinal malignant diseases; in occasional patients with nonmalignant hepatic disease where active hepatic regeneration was occurring; and in a few patients with nongastrointestinal malignant disorders metastatic to the liver.[1,10]

The metabolic half-life of AFP has been determined to be approximately 5 days.[11] These determinations, however, were made in healthy humans; the metabolic clearance of AFP in patients with cancer or in the postoperative period is not known, although calculations using the 5-day figure seem to be accurate clinically (P. H. Lange, unpublished data). A number of investigations using histochemical techniques have determined that the cell type that is responsible for AFP production in testicular tumor morphologically resembles yolk sac tissue. Thus the presence of AFP in the serum of a testicular tumor patient has been attributed to foci of yolk sac differentiation even in tumors where such foci are undetected and the tumor is otherwise designated as embryonal cell carcinoma or teratocarcinoma.[12] However, the histochemical techniques for AFP cellular localization are still being improved and it is probable that the morphological characterization of the cell type that secretes AFP in NSGCT will be redefined.

Human chorionic gonadotropin is a glycoprotein of approximately 38,000 molecular weight which normally is secreted by specialized cells in the human placenta. It is composed of two dissimilar polypeptide chains designated alpha and beta. The alpha subunit is similar to the alpha subunit of the pituitary glycoprotein hormones, luteinizing hormone (LH), follicle-stimulating hormone (FSH), and thyrotropic stimulating hormone (TSH). The beta subunit of hCG, however, is much less similar to that of the beta subunits of LH, FSH, and TSH, particularly in its terminal 29 amino acids. Thus some antibodies produced in laboratory animals against purified hCG beta subunits may cross-react very little with physiologic concentrations of LH. Radioimmunoassays using such antibodies can thus be made very sensitive (less than 1 ng/ml) and very specific for the whole hCG molecule or for its freely circulating beta subunit.[8,13] It is important to realize, however, that cross-reactivity with LH will vary considerably among various beta-hCG assays depending on the particular antibody used, and the physician must exercise caution when low abnormal or borderline abnormal levels of hCG are recorded using these assays (*vide infra*).

It has, of course, been known for some time that hCG is found in the sera of some patients with germ cell tumors containing trophoblastic elements. With the development of sensitive beta-chain hCG radioimmunoassays, the incidence of NSGCT patients with hCG in their serum increased to 40–60%. Using radioimmunoassays, hCG has also been detected in the sera of a wide variety of cancers including liver, breast, stomach, pancreas, and lung.[8] More recently, it was appreciated that some patients with pure seminoma also have abnormal hCG levels in their serum (*vide infra*).

Gestational trophoblastic tumors and other human neoplasms that are associated with hCG production do not always secrete the whole molecule. Some tumors produce free alpha or beta hCG chains exclusively or in unbalanced fashion, while others may manufacture abnormal molecular forms of hCG and its subunits.[14,15] The metabolic half-life of the whole hCG molecule is approximately 30 hr.[16] However, the subunits have much shorter half-lives: 20 min for the alpha chain and 45 min for the beta chain.[13] It is probable that testicular tumors also differ in their secretion of whole, subunit, or abnormal hCG molecules.

Specificity and Incidence of AFP/hCG in Testicular Tumor

To be clinically effective in testicular tumor, AFP and hCG must not only be measured by sensitive assays, but they must be measured together. This is because approximately 40% of patients with NSGCT have an elevation of only one marker[2] and because, in the clinical course of the disease, the markers do not always parallel each other. For example, the level of one marker may fall with therapy while the other does not fall or may actually rise.[17] Alternatively, the level of one marker may be normal initially only to rise later during treatment while the other marker falls to normal levels.

However, when measured together, AFP and hCG are very prevalent in testicular tumor. Reported figures have varied from 59 to 91%[1,3,18]; our current incidence is 84% among 275 patients who had active disease at the time of serum determinations. This figure, while impressive, is misleading because the incidence of marker elevations in NSGCT patients varies greatly with the stage of the disease. In addition, the frequency of elevated markers in seminoma is much lower (*vide infra*).

As previously discussed, both markers are occasionally elevated in a variety of malignant diseases and even in some nonmalignant states. However, our experience has shown that in patients thought or known to have testicular tumor, these markers are, in a practical sense, very specific for testicular tumor, especially NSGCT. We have yet to see an elevated marker in testicular tumor patients that was due to any of the other pathological states that can cause elevations of these markers. Moreover, even if such an event should occur, we feel that these other causes for elevated markers can be ruled out during routine clinical evaluation.

Perhaps more important, there have been no true false-positive marker determinations reported in testicular tumor patients (that is, the situation where a marker is truly elevated and yet the patient has no disease at the time of the marker determination or subsequently). There are two caveats to this principle, however. One is that a marker may be elevated in a tumor-free patient because the substance has not yet been metabolically cleared, as may occur within several days after orchiectomy in a Stage I NSGCT patient. The other caveat is that very low elevations of hCG may occasionally be recorded in patients who actually have only elevated LH serum levels. This event usually has occurred when one of the less-specific commercial beta-hCG assays is used, but it can occur even with some highly specific hCG assays when the patient's serum LH level is especially high. This phenomenon is relevant to the testicular tumor patient since he may have elevated LH levels because he has been rendered hypogonadal by chemotherapy and/or orchiectomy. However, when reliable radioimmunoassays are used, these false hCG elevations are rare and usually only borderline abnormal. If necessary, short-term administration of testosterone to the patient and then retesting will resolve the issue.[19]

Preoperative Value of AFP and hCG

Our current figures on the preoperative value of serum markers in testicular tumor are given in Table I. Certainly determinations of AFP and hCG before the exploration of a scrotal mass are of limited value. Normal marker levels are always seen in patients with benign scrotal masses, but normal preoperative levels are also observed in approximately one-third of the patients with Stage I NSGCT and a majority of patients with seminoma regardless of stage. Thus AFP and hCG levels are of value in the differential diagnosis of scrotal masses only if the levels are abnormal, in which case the clinician can be reasonably certain that the patient has a testicular tumor.

Table I.

Value of Preoperative AFP and HCG

	Before orchiectomy				Before retroperitoneal lymphadenectomy for NSGCT		
Diagnosis	No. of pts.	Elevated AFP or hCG +	−	Diagnosis	No. of pts.	Elevated AFP or hCG +	−
Benign scrotal masses	37	0	37	NSGCT			
Seminoma	37	6	31	Stage I	37	2[a]	35
NSGCT				Stage II	29	21	8
Stage I	30	20	10				
Stage II or greater	28	26	2				

[a] Stage II, serologic only.

The value of determining marker levels in NSGCT patients before they have retroperitoneal lymphadenectomy also requires clarification. For example, a working knowledge of the metabolic clearance of these markers is often necessary. This is more true for AFP with its longer half-life than it is for hCG. In many circumstances, particularly before and after lymphadenectomy, a single elevated marker value cannot be used to determine the presence of metastasis because it could reflect either the continued presence of tumor or a normally falling serum titer after removal of all marker-producing neoplasm. However, if at least two values taken several days apart are available, one can calculate the expected value by constructing a curve or from the following equations:

$$\text{for hCG:} \quad X_F = X_0 e^{-0.023(th)},$$

$$\text{for AFP:} \quad X_F = X_0 e^{-0.139(td)},$$

where X_0 is the initial marker concentration and X_F is the concentration at time t in days (d) or in hours (h). Parenthetically, one should take into account the effects of blood transfusions and possibly the metabolic effects of surgery when interpreting marker clearance data.

But even when metabolic decay is accounted for, there are a significant number of patients who have pathologically proven retroperitoneal metastases and normal preoperative marker levels. The exact frequency of these "false negatives" varies depending on the series but will probably settle around 20–40%. In many of the cases, though by no means all, these false negatives occur in patients who only have microscopic retroperitoneal metastases. However, a more important concern is the accuracy of preoperative staging when marker determinations are combined with lymphangiography or the newer techniques of computerized tomography and abdominal echography. This problem is still incompletely resolved. In our series and that of Scardino,[3] the staging error is certainly diminished when marker levels are added to the other staging modalities, but it is still significant (10–25%). Also, marker determinations cannot be used in lieu of other staging procedures because there are instances where the marker levels are normal while the other diagnostic modalities correctly diagnose retroperitoneal metastasis.

From the aforementioned facts, it is apparent that some primary or metastatic NSGCT tumors do not cause elevated serum marker levels. However, it has been suggested that if the primary NSGCT tumor in the scrotum is shown to produce markers (e.g., the marker levels are elevated before or immediately after orchiectomy) and the levels return to normal after surgery, then one can assume that there are no retroperitoneal metastases and possibly avoid lymphadenectomy. In our view, such a protocol would be ill advised. We have seen a significant number of patients who were marker-positive before orchiectomy, whose markers returned to normal after orchiectomy, and yet who were found to have metastatic NSGCT. Clearly currently available noninvasive staging methods including AFP/hCG determinations should not be used to decide against lymphadenectomy. On the other hand, false-positive marker levels before lymphadenectomy have not occurred, so any patient with elevated markers before lymphadenectomy, unless these can be explained by the rate of metabolic decay, should be considered to have metastatic disease. Clearly retroperitoneal lymphadenectomy is still the best staging technique.

If retroperitoneal lymphadenectomy should be done regardless of the marker levels, why then should marker levels be determined before such surgery? The answer to this question requires further study, but at present we believe that preoperative marker determinations should be obtained for the following reasons:

1. If the preoperative and immediately postoperative values are known, one may diagnose unappreciated persistent disease earlier. Moreover, since many

of the patients who might have persistent disease (e.g., those with gross evidence of retroperitoneal lymph node involvement at surgery) are now being treated with postoperative chemotherapy, it would be important to know if such treatment was being administered as adjuvant or active therapy.

2. We have observed a phenomenon which we call "Stage II disease, serologic only." That is, pre-lymphadenectomy marker levels are truly elevated and not due to the metabolic clearance considerations, the pathologist even after repeated examination can find no metastatic disease in the resected retroperitoneal lymph nodes, and yet the marker levels fall after surgery according to metabolic decay rates thereby confirming that marker-producing tumor was removed. These cases may fall into a separate prognostic group.

3. A knowledge of whether a tumor does or does not produce elevated serum marker levels may have prognostic significance (vide infra).

4. Advances in staging techniques and new or more sensitive tumor markers (vide infra) may increase the possibility that noninvasive methods of staging will ultimately prove reliable. Continued collection of preoperative AFP/hCG marker data will facilitate this possibility.

Serial Monitoring of NSGCT Patients after Initial Treatment(s)

The greatest value of accurate AFP and hCG determinations in testicular tumor is in the follow-up of patients with Stage I and Stage II NSGCT after surgery or in monitoring the effectiveness of chemotherapy in patients with advanced disease. There are many published case reports that illustrate the clinical usefulness of these markers.[2,3,13,17,18,20-23] We have now followed 173 NSGCT patients with marker determinations from the time of their initial active disease for as long as 35 months. The following are some of the conclusions that we have made on the basis of this experience:

The marker values usually reflect or predict, sometimes by as much as 6 months, the progression or remission of disease. There have been no false positive values in patients known or later confirmed to be free of disease provided one accounts for the metabolic clearance and the problems of LH cross-reactivity as previously discussed. Moreover, the use of serial markers should not be restricted to patients with known metastatic disease on chemotherapy or to patients at high risk for recurrence (e.g., Stage II disease with bulky metastasis). For example, we have been alerted to tumor recurrence after lymphadenectomy by marker levels in patients who had Stage I NSGCT. In fact today we would begin chemotherapy in a NSGCT patient who had elevated marker levels after his initial surgery(s) without a pathologic confirmation in those situations where to do so would require major surgery.

In NSGCT patients when both AFP and hCG are normal despite clinical evidence of persistent or growing masses, the diagnosis may be benign disease (e.g., mesenteric cyst, lymphocele), pure seminoma, or adult teratoma. False negative marker values do occur in Stage III patients (i.e., the patient has active metastatic disease with normal AFP and hCG levels), but these events are not common. Among 125 of our patients who had Stage III disease and who were followed with serial marker levels, 13 (10%) had active NSGCT at the time of the negative marker levels. These "false negatives" are of several types:

1. the patient is always marker negative from the onset of his disease;
2. the patient is marker positive at the time of his initial tumor but is negative at the time of tumor recurrence or persistently active disease; or
3. the patient's abnormal marker levels decline to normal yet clinical evidence of disease regresses more slowly but also eventually disappears as chemotherapy continues (the so-called "lag phenomenon").

In eight of nine of these falsely negative Stage III patients in whom adequate clinical follow-up was available, complete remission was very quickly achieved with chemotherapy. This leads us to speculate that such falsely negative tumors may have a particularly good prognosis.

Therefore, we continue to suggest that AFP and hCG serum determinations are indispensible in monitoring testicular tumor patients. Furthermore, patients with Stage III disease who previously had elevated serum marker levels and who later demonstrate persistently normal AFP and hCG despite continued or enlarging masses, should have surgical biopsy before the initiation or continuation of chemotherapy.

Prognostic Value of Marker Levels

There is a definite correlation between stage of disease and the presence in the serum of elevation AFP and/or hCG. In our present series 66% of Stage I disease and 93% of Stage II or greater disease had elevated markers before orchiectomy. Thus, as disease becomes more extensive, the markers are more frequently elevated. In this sense, there is a correlation between marker status and prognosis. However, are serum marker levels merely a reflection of the bulk of the disease and therefore only a commentary on disease stage, or is the fact that a NSGCT tumor produces elevated serum markers an indication of its potential or actual aggressiveness regardless of bulk or stage of disease at the time of presentation? Comparison of serum markers in patients with equal stage and bulk of disease are needed to explore this question. Data on such a comparison are not published, although it has been suggested that AFP/hCG levels may be an independent prognostic variable.[3] Other evidence substantiating such a theory includes the fact that tumors containing only adult teratoma rarely have elevated marker levels and our suspicion that falsely negative Stage III patients may respond particularly well to chemotherapy.

AFP and hCG in Seminoma

Recently it has become apparent that patients with a diagnosis of pure seminoma do occasionally have elevated marker levels.[2,24] We recently completed a case analysis of 31 patients who exhibited this phenomenon.[25] While a definite statement about the meaning and therapy of such patients will require completion of a controlled prospective study, our tentative conclusions are as follows:

1. Serum marker levels should be serially determined on all patients with seminoma.
2. If the AFP is elevated, this is irrefutable evidence for the existence of NSGCT, and the patient should be treated accordingly even without pathological documentation.
3. If only the hCG level is elevated, the patient could have the simultaneous presence of NSGCT, but the hCG level is also consistent with what, after extensive clinical analysis, still appears to be pure seminoma. Parenthetically the exact incidence of elevated hCG in seminoma is still unclear but probably will be about 5–10% in studies involving unbiased populations.
4. In a seminoma patient with an elevated hCG level, one should make every attempt to be sure that he truly has pure seminoma.
5. Patients with pure seminoma and elevated hCG levels do respond to radiation therapy particularly if the disease is of low stage.
6. Elevated hCG levels, however, may predict those patients who will not respond well to radiation therapy, particularly if the disease is of the higher stages. These patients, however, do appear to respond well to chemotherapy.

The Future

The fortuitous availability of sensitive radioimmunoassays for AFP and hCG at a time when major advances were occurring in the chemotherapy of testicular tumor provided a poignant example of the ability of sensitive tumor markers to influence the care of the tumor patient. Yet even in the field of testicular tumor, the era of tumor markers is only beginning. First of all there are many clinical aspects about the meaning of AFP/hCG levels that need further clarification; some of these have been discussed in this article. Another possible clinical use of the markers is to predict the response to chemotherapy using the phenomenon of "apparent half-life." That is, the marker levels of some patients undergoing the induction phase of chemotherapy decline at a rate similar to the theoretical metabolic clearance of those markers assuming no further production by the tumor, while the markers of other patients decline much slower, although they may also eventually become normal. Our preliminary experience[26] and that of others[27,28] suggests that a comparison of the actual marker decay curve with the theoretical curve may be used to predict the eventual response to chemotherapy within the first several weeks after induction.

It is also probable that there will be increasingly sensitive methods for measuring hCG. For example, using special urine concentrating techniques and a more specific beta-hCG assay, the sensitivity of hCG determinations can be greatly increased.[29] The value of this technique in monitoring testicular tumor patients, especially those patients whose marker levels have declined toward normal with therapy, is currently under study.[13]

An analysis of the molecular heterogeneity of hCG and possibly AFP may someday provide additional important clinical information. As previously discussed, it is apparent that some tumors can secrete intact hCG molecules or free alpha or beta chains in various proportions. In gestational trophoblastic tumors a characterization of these proportions seems to have prognostic significance. There is also evidence in animals that tumors can produce different varieties of AFP,[30] and it may be that the same is true in man. Investigations into the molecular hetereogeneity of AFP and hCG are now being conducted in human testicular tumor.

It is probable that in the future other tumor markers will be useful clinically in testicular tumor. For example, experimental studies are revealing a whole host of new oncodevelopmental antigens. These antigens, of which carcinoembryonic antigen (CEA), AFP, and hCG are examples, are defined as substances which appear temporarily in the course of normal embryological development, disappear as ontogenesis progresses, but then may be produced anew during the course of oncogenesis. One such new antigen, which seems important in testicular tumor, is Pregnancy Specific Beta-$_1$Glycoprotein (or SP-1). This antigen, which is only one of many putative specific placental proteins, is found in the sera of normal pregnant women but also in the sera of patients with trophoblastic tumors and NSGCT.[31] Our preliminary studies using a sensitive radioimmunoassay suggest that SP-1 is a useful additional tumor marker in testicular tumor.[32]

Similarly experimental studies on the murine teratocarcinoma model have revealed other oncodevelopmental antigens.[33] One group of antigens, called the F9 antigens, have been demonstrated on human NSGCT tissue cultured cells[34] and probably on the cells of fresh NSGCT also (P. H. Lange, unpublished data). Whether this group of antigens will have clinical importance is unexplored at present.

There is evidence that the clinically well-traveled serum enzyme lactic dehydrogenase (LDH) may be an additional useful tumor marker in testicular tumor patients.[35–37] In our studies, LDH was elevated in 63% of patients, but, more importantly, the addition of LDH determinations to those of AFP and hCG increased the percentage of testicular tumor patients with positive serum markers from 86% to 93%.[38] LDH is, of course, not specific for testicular tumor and its true value in the monitoring of such patients remains to be defined.

It is hoped that oncodevelopmental antigens can be used to localize metastases either by radioactive scanning techniques or by measuring marker gradients within blood vessels. Javadpour and his group succeeded in localizing a metastatic testicular tumor using blood vessel catheterization studies for the alpha chain of hCG. However, as very elegantly described by these investigators, this technique probably will have limited application.[23] Likewise the use of radioisotope techniques has not yet achieved the level of clinical fruition mainly because of technical problems related to background activity. Some progress has been made recently with CEA,[39] and several groups are currently working on such techniques for AFP and hCG.

Histochemical analysis of testicular tumor tissue for AFP and hCG has been accomplished by many investigators,[12,40-42] although technical problems particularly with AFP have hindered progress. It is already apparent, however, that many of our concepts about the cellular histology and even the origin of NSGCT may be altered by these studies. Furthermore, histochemical cellular analysis for other oncodevelopmental antigens is only now beginning in testicular tumor. Finally a simplified method for measuring the concentration of AFP within the tumor itself has been developed.[43] It is entirely possible that the analysis of tumor marker content and cellular localization will have significant prognostic or therapeutic value and may become a routine part of the pathological analysis of testicular tumors in the future.

Lastly, at a more basic level, the oncodevelopmental antigens have provided investigators with models for examining more closely the mechanisms of gene expression. For example, human tissue-cultured cell lines that can produce hCG, its alpha-chain, or beta-chain are available, and factors which "turn on" and "turn off" marker production within these cells have been discovered.[44-46] These experimental models may allow scientists to reveal how the genes responsible for marker production are activated and later repressed in the normal situation, how embryological development occurs at the molecular level, and possibly also something about the mechanisms responsible for abnormal gene expression as may occur in neoplasia.

References

1. Waldmann, T. A., and McIntire, K. R.: The use of radioimmunoassay for alpha-fetoprotein in the diagnosis of malignancy. *Cancer* **34**:1510–1515, 1974.

2. Lange, P. H., and Fraley, E. E.: Serum alpha-fetoprotein and human chorionic gonadotropin in the treatment of patients with testicular tumors. *Urol Clin North Am* **4**:393–406, 1977.

3. Scardino, P. T., Cox, H. D., Waldmann, T. A., *et al.*: The value of serum tumor markers in the staging and prognosis of germ cell tumors of the testis. *J Urol* **118**:994–999, 1977.

4. Waldmann, T. A., and McIntire, K. R.: Serum alpha-fetoprotein levels in patients with ataxia-telangiectasia. *Lancet* **2**:1112–1115, 1971.

5. Vaitukaitis, J. L., Braunstein, G. D., and Ross, G. T.: A radioimmunoassay which specifically measures human chorionic gonadotropin in the presence of human luteinizing hormone. *Am J Obstet Gynecol* **113**:751–758, 1972.

6. Vessella, R. L., Lange, P. H., and Simon, F.: The development of a sensitive radioimmunoassay for AFP. (submitted for publication).

7. Nørgaard-Pedersen, B.: Human alpha-fetoprotein. *Scand J Immunol Suppl* #4, 1976.

8. Vaitukaitis, J. L., Ross, G. T., Braunstein, G. D., et al.: Gonadotropins and their subunits. Basic and clinical studies. *Recent Prog Horm Res* **32**:289–331, 1976.

9. Fishman, W. H., and Sell, S.: San Diego Conference on Oncodevelopmental Gene Expression (meeting report) *Cancer Res* **36**:3856–3858, 1976.

10. Grenier, A., Laberge, C., Valet, J. P., et al.: Neonatal mass screening of hereditary tyrosinemia with blood alpha-1-fetoprotein. *Carcino-Embryonic Proteins*, Vol. 2. Lehmann, F. G. (Ed.). Elsevier/North-Holland Biomedical Press 1979, pp. 425–433.

11. Gitlin, D., and Boesman, M.: Serum alpha-fetoprotein, albumin, and gammaglobulin in the human conceptus. *J Clin Invest* **45**:1826–1838, 1966.

12. Nørgaard-Pedersen, B., Albrechtsen, R., and Teilum, G.: Serum alpha-fetoprotein as a marker for endodermal sinus tumor (yolk sac tumour) or a vitelline component of "teratocarcinoma." *Acta Pathol Microbiol Scand* (A) **83**:573–589, 1975.

13. Javadpour, N.: The National Cancer Institute's experience with testicular cancer. *J Urol* **120**:651–659, 1978.

14. Kahn, C. R., Rosen, S. W., Weintraub, B. D., et al.: Ectopic production of chorionic gonadotropin and its subunits by islet-cell tumors. *N Engl J Med* **297**:565–569, 1977.

15. Vaitukaitis, J. L., and Ebersole, E. R.: Evidence of altered synthesis of human chorionic gonadotropin in gestational trophoblastic tumors. *J Clin Endocrinol Metab* **42**:1048–1055, 1976.

16. Rizhallah, T., Grupide, E., and VandeWiele, R.: Metabolism of hCG in man. *J Clin Endocrinol* **29**:92–100, 1969.

17. Braunstein, G. D., McIntire, K. R., and Waldmann, T. A.: Discordance of human chorionic gonadotropin and alpha-fetoprotein in testicular teratocarcinomas. *Cancer* **31**:1065–1068, 1973.

18. Schultz, H., Sell, A., Nørgaard-Pedersen, B., et al.: Serum alpha-fetoprotein and human chorionic gonadotropin as markers for the effect of postoperative radiation therapy and/or chemotherapy in testicular cancer. *Cancer* **42**:2182–2186, 1978.

19. Catalona, W. J., Vaitukaitis, J. L., and Fair, W. R.: Falsely positive specific human chorionic gonadotropin assays in patients with testicular tumors. Conversion to negative with testosterone administration. *J Urol* **122**:126–128, 1979.

20. Perlin, E., Engeler, J. E., Jr., Edson, M., et al.: The value of serial measurement of both human chorionic gonadotropin and alpha-fetoprotein for monitoring germinal cell tumors. *Cancer* **37**:215–219, 1976.

21. Lange, P. H.: Serum alpha-fetoprotein and human chorionic gonadotropin in the management of testicular tumors. *Natl Cancer Inst Monogr* **49**:215–217, 1978.

22. Lange, P. H., McIntire, K. R., Waldmann, T. A., et al.: Serum alpha-fetoprotein and human chorionic gonadotropin in the diagnosis and management of nonseminomatous germ-cell testicular cancer. *N Engl J Med* **295**:1237–1240, 1976.

23. Javadpour, N., McIntire, K. R., Waldmann, T. A., et al.: The role of the radioimmunoassay of serum alpha-fetoprotein and human chorionic gonadotropin in the intensive chemotherapy and surgery of metastatic testicular tumors. *J Urol* **119**:759–762, 1978.

24. Javadpour, N., McIntire, K. R., and Waldmann, T. A.: Human chorionic gonadotropin (HCG) and alpha-fetoprotein (AFP) in sera and tumor cells of patients with testicular seminoma. *Cancer* **42**:2768–2772, 1978.

25. Lange, P. H., Nochomovitz, L., E., Rosai, J., et al.: Serum alpha-fetoprotein and human chorionic gonadotropin in patients with seminoma. *J Urol* (in press).

26. Lange, P. H., Bosl, G. J., Kennedy, B. J., et al.: Marker decay curves in testicular tumor—a prognostic tool. (submitted for publication).

27. Kohn, J.: The value of apparent half-life assay of AFP in the management of teratoma. Recent Progress. *Carcino-Embryonic Proteins*, Volume 2. Lehmann, F. G. (Ed.). Elsevier/North-Holland Biomedical Press 1979.

28. Thompson, D. K., Haddow, J. E., and Ritchie, R. F.: Serial monitoring of serum AFP and beta-hCG in germ cell tumors. Recent Progress. *Carcino-Embryonic Proteins*, Vol. 2. Lehmann, F. G. (Ed.). Elsevier/North-Holland Biomedical Press 1979.

29. Ayala, A. R., Nisula, B. C., Chen, H. C., *et al.*: Highly sensitive radioimmunoassay for chorionic gonadotropin in human urine. *J Clin Endocrinol Metab* **47**:767–773, 1978.

30. Smith, C. J., Morris, H. P., and Kelleher, P. C.: Concanavalin A affinity molecular variance of alpha-fetoprotein in neonatal rat serum and in the serum of rats bearing hepatomas. *Cancer Res* **37**:2651–2656, 1977.

31. Horne, C. H. W., and Towler, C. M.: Pregnancy-specific β_1-glycoprotein: A review. *Obstet Gynecol Surv* **33**:761–768, 1978.

32. Lange, P. H., Bremner, R. D., Horne, C. H. W., *et al.*: Is SP-1 a marker for testicular cancer? (submitted for publication).

33. Gachelin, G.: The cell surface antigens of mouse embryonal carcinoma cells. *Biochim Biophys Acta* **516**:27–60, 1978.

34. Solter, D., and Knowles, B. B.: Monoclonal antibody defining a stage-specific mouse embryonic antigen (SSEA-1). *Proc Natl Acad Sci USA* **75**:5565–5569, 1978.

35. Boyle, L. E., and Samuels, M. L.: Serum LDH activity and isoenzyme patterns in non-seminomatous germinal (NSG) testis tumors. *Proc Am Assoc Clin Oncol* **18**:278, 1977 (Abstract #C-48).

36. VonEyben, F. E.: Biochemical markers in advanced testicular tumors—serum lactate dehydrogenase, urinary chorionic gonadotropin, and total urinary estrogens. *Cancer* **41**:648–652, 1978.

37. Cheng, E., Cvitkovic, E., Wittes, R. E., *et al.*: Germ cell tumors (II). VABII in metastatic testicular cancer. *Cancer* **42**:2162–2168, 1978.

38. Bosl, G. J., Lange, P. H., Nochomovitz, L., *et al.*: Biologic markers in advanced testis cancer. (submitted for publication).

39. Goldenberg, D. N., Primus, F. J., Kim, E., *et al.*: Radioimmune detection of cancer in man: The use of radiolabeled antibodies to CEA. Recent Progress. *Carcino-Embryonic Proteins*, Volume 2. Lehmann, F. G. (Ed.). Elsevier/North-Holland Biomedical Press 1979.

40. Palmer, P. E., Safaii, H., and Wolfe, H. J.: Alpha$_1$-antitrypsin and alpha-fetoprotein: Protein markers in endodermal sinus (yolk sac) tumors. *Am J Clin Pathol* **65**:575–582, 1976.

41. Kurman, R. J., Scardino, P. T., McIntire, K. R., *et al.*: Cellular localization of alpha-fetoprotein and human chorionic gonadotropin in germ cell tumors of the testis using an indirect immunoperoxidase technique. A new approach to classification utilizing tumor markers. *Cancer* **40**:2136–2151, 1977.

42. Heyderman, E.: Multiple tissue markers in human malignant testicular tumours. *Carcinoembryonic Proteins*. Nørgaard-Pedersen, B. and Axelsen, N. H. (Eds.). *Recent Prog Suppl Scand J Immunol* No. 8, 1978.

43. Nørgaard-Pedersen, B., Albrechtsen, R., Hagerstrand, I., *et al.*: Tumor markers in gonadal and extragonadal germ cell tumors. Recent Progress. *Carcino-Embryonic Proteins*, Volume 2. Lehmann, F. G. (Ed.). Elsevier/North Holland Biomedical Press 1979.

44. Hussa, R. O., and Story, M. T.: Tumor antigen and human chorionic gonadotropin CaSki cells. A new epidermoid cervical cancer cell line. *Science* **196**:1456–1458, 1977.

45. Ghosh, N. K., and Cox, R. P.: Production of human chorionic gonadotropin in HeLa cell culture. *Nature* **259**:416–417, 1976.

46. Lieblick, J. M., Weintraub, B. D., Rosen, S. W., *et al.*: Secretion of hCG alpha subunit and hCG by HeLa strains. *Nature* **265**:746, 1977.

5

Abdominal Ultrasound and Computed Tomography in Testicular Cancer

Bryan T. Burney, M.D. and Eugene C. Klatte, M.D.

Department of Radiology, Indiana University Medical Center, Indianapolis, Indiana

Introduction

AGGRESSIVE SURGICAL and combination chemotherapy approaches have produced a disease-free state in large numbers of patients with disseminated testicular cancers.[1] Management of these patients requires repeated evaluation of chest and abdominal disease. Usually this is accomplished with chest radiographs and whole lung tomography above the diaphragm and intravenous pyelography and bipedal lymphangiography below the diaphragm.

Ultrasound[2–4] and computed tomography[5,6] are ideal for imaging the abdomen and retroperitoneal space and both have proved useful in staging lymphomas.[7–10] In a similar fashion both modalities are useful for imaging lymph nodes enlarged with metastatic testicular cancer in the retroperitoneal space. In addition ultrasound and computed tomography provide information about the other abdominal

83

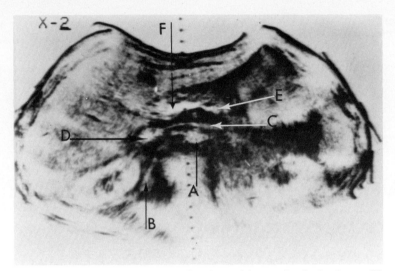

FIGURE 1A. Ultrasound cross section shows aorta (a), crus of right diaphragm (b), left renal vein (c), entering the inferior vena cava (d). The splenic vein (e), and portal vein (f), are also shown.

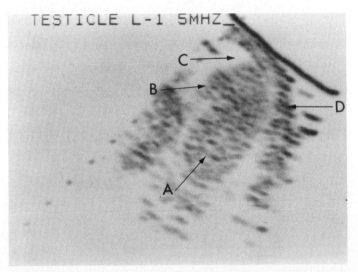

FIGURE 1B. A normal testicle (a), with epididymis (b), and a small hydrocele (c), is shown on a parasagittal ultrasound section. The scrotum (d) can also be seen.

organs and soft tissues. At least some of this information cannot be obtained by any other method short of laparotomy. This chapter is based on experience during a 2-year period with over 300 abdominal ultrasound examinations and over 200

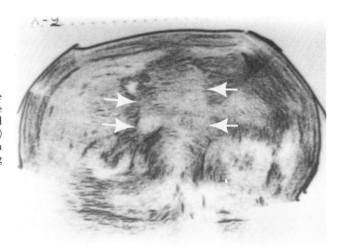

FIGURE 2A. The middle portion of the abdomen is obscured by artifacts (arrows) produced from bowel gas overlying the area.

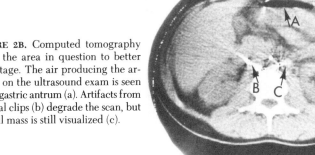

FIGURE 2B. Computed tomography shows the area in question to better advantage. The air producing the artifacts on the ultrasound exam is seen in the gastric antrum (a). Artifacts from surgical clips (b) degrade the scan, but a small mass is still visualized (c).

abdominal computed tomography examinations in 140 patients with prior orchiectomies for carcinoma of the testicle.

Advantages and Disadvantages

Ultrasound uses high frequency (1–5 MHz) sound waves to produce cross-sectional and sagittal images of the abdomen (Fig. 1). The sound beam intensities used for diagnostic imaging cause no harmful effect, so ultrasound examinations may be repeated as frequently as necessary. The quality of the image obtained is as much dependent on the skill of the ultrasonographer as it is on the quality of the equipment used. Significant degradation of ultrasound scans is caused by

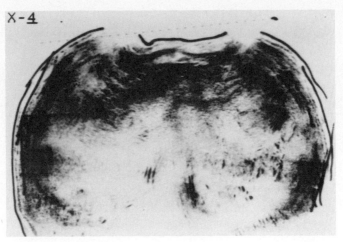

FIGURE 3A. Ultrasound examination of this obese patient was futile.

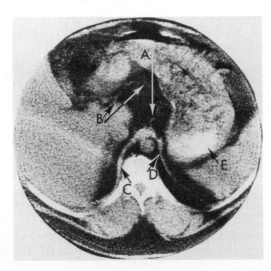

FIGURE 3B. A computed tomography section at the same level in the same patient outlines the celiac axis (a), the common hepatic artery (b), and the crurae of the diaphragm (c and d). Radiopaque iodinated contrast material is layered posteriorly in the gastric fundus (e).

bowel gas which reflects the sound beam and causes severe artifacts (Fig. 2). Because of this, ultrasound examinations should be performed prior to administration of chemotherapy, which can cause nausea and accumulation of excessive gas in the bowel.

The ultrasound beam is attenuated rapidly as it passes through large masses of soft tissue. For this reason, obese patients are not good candidates for ultrasound examination (Fig. 3). Fresh barium sulfate in the bowel also causes reflection of the sound beam similar to that caused by bowel gas (Fig. 4). Underlying structures are shielded from view. Barium that has been in the bowel for several days presents somewhat less of a problem, although it can easily be mistaken for an echogenic mass.

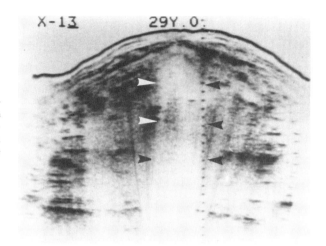

FIGURE 4A. The discrete shadow (arrows) on the ultrasound examination is due to fesh barium in the transverse colon.

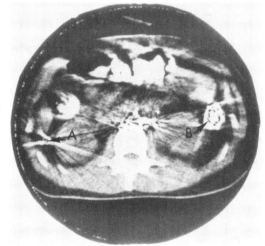

FIGURE 4B. Artifacts from the extremely radiopaque barium are best seen surrounding barium in the ascending colon (a) and as spurious low density areas within the descending colon (b).

Computed tomography detects differences as small as 0.1% in the attenuation of x-ray photons by adjacent tissues to produce a cross-sectional image. The obese patient is an ideal candidate for computed tomography because fat provides a low density contrast medium that neatly outlines internal structures (Fig. 5). However, in the patient without significant amounts of body fat, especially when due to chronic illness, tissue plains are very poorly defined by computed tomography (Fig. 6). In these cases excellent, highly diagnostic images can usually be obtained by ultrasound. When triaging patients between examinations it is a good rule of thumb to send the skinny patients to ultrasound and the fat patients to computed tomography.

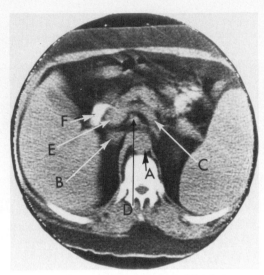

FIGURE 5. Fat neatly outlines the aorta (a), inferior vena cava (b), the splenic vein (c), and the superior mesenteric artery (d). The portal vein superior mesenteric vein splenic vein confluence (e) can be seen causing an impression on the descending duodenum (f), which is filled with orally administrated iodinated contrast material.

Computed tomography scanning times vary with the equipment in use. Scanning times in the 2–20-sec range are the rule in most hospitals. Any patient or bowel gas motion during this time significantly degrades the scan. Patients who are unable to suspend respiration for the full length of the scan are probably better imaged by ultrasound. Glucagon may be administered (0.5 mg intravenously) to decrease artifact production from active peristalsis in those patients with large amounts of bowel gas.[11] Barium in the bowel will frequently degrade the scan significantly.

Metallic surgical clips placed during retroperitoneal node dissection produce stellate artifacts that make computed tomography scans uninterpretable (Fig. 7). It has been reported that changing to surgical clips made of titanium reduces artifact production.[12]

Fluid has no acoustic interfaces to produce echoes. For this reason fluid is detected more readily by ultrasound than by computed tomography. Cystic changes in masses, small amounts of ascites (Fig. 8), and renal obstruction (Fig. 9) are usually detected more easily with ultrasound than with computed tomography. Of course, computed tomography can be used to diagnose all of these entities.

The ability of ultrasound to produce sagittal (longitudinal) images provides an advantage over computed tomography in some cases (Figs. 10–12).

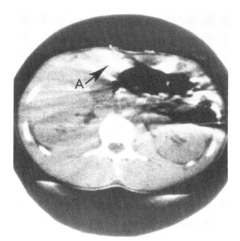

FIGURE 6A. A patient without a significant amount of retroperitoneal fat is a poor candidate for computed tomography. Normal anatomical landmarks are not identifiable. Peristaltic motion of bowel containing air produces opaque artifacts (a), which also degrade the scan.

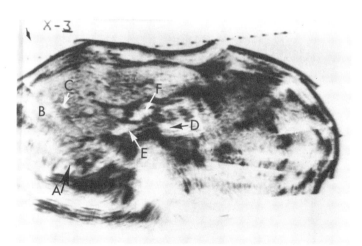

FIGURE 6B. An ultrasound section in the same patient at the same level easily shows the kidney (a) and liver (b), with small hepatic veins (c). The aorta (d), inferior vena cava (e), and portal vein (f) are also clearly seen.

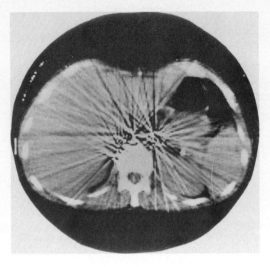

FIGURE 7A. Metallic clips placed during previous retroperitoneal lymph node dissection render this computed tomography slice uninterpretable.

Patient Preparation and Performance of Scans

Ultrasound examination requires no advance patient preparation. The less bowel gas the better, so examinations should be performed prior to administration of chemotherapy. Making the patient NPO after midnight prior to the examination may be useful in some instances. Simethicone has not proved useful in our

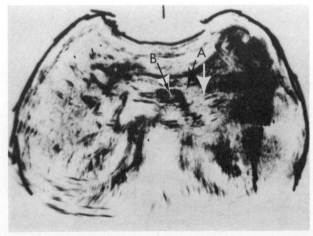

FIGURE 7B. In contrast, an ultrasound section at the same level in the same patient shows normal anatomy including the pancreas (a) and the superior mesenteric artery (b).

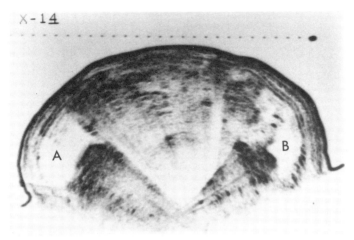
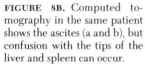

FIGURE 8A. Ascites in both flanks (a) and (b) is easily detected with ultrasound.

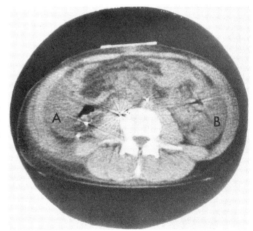

FIGURE 8B. Computed tomography in the same patient shows the ascites (a and b), but confusion with the tips of the liver and spleen can occur.

experience. In some instances a repeat exam on another day may be necessary if gas artifacts are excessive.

No medications need to be administered for an ultrasound examination. Charges for an ultrasound examination are usually at least 50% lower than charges for abdominal computed tomography.

Computed tomography also requires no advance patient preparation. However, radiographic contrast medications must be administered to the patient during the scan in many cases. Branching portal veins in the liver can simulate metastatic lesions unless they are opacified with high doses of intravenously administered

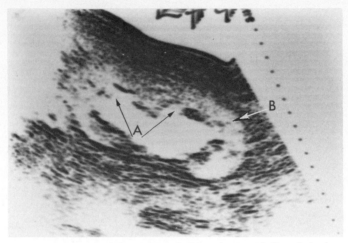

FIGURE 9A. Ultrasound demonstrates hydronephrosis with distended calyces (a) and normal cortex (b).

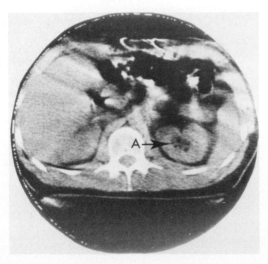

FIGURE 9B. Low density fat (a) in the renal pelvis of a normal kidney can be mistaken for hydronephrosis in which urine (water density) occupies the central portion of the kidney.

iodinated contrast agents such as sodium diatrizoate (Fig. 13). Low-density fat in the renal pelvis can be confused with hydronephrosis unless the renal collecting systems are opacified.

Normally, iodinated contrast agents are freely administered, but patients with dissemminated testicular cancer are frequently receiving cis-diamminedichloro platinum. Platinum is nephrotoxic, and iodinated contrast media can be ne-

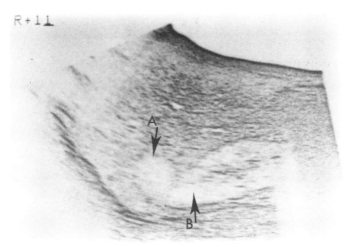

FIGURE 10A. Metastatic embryonal cell carcinoma (a) is seen in the liver above the upper pole of the right kidney (b), on a parasagittal ultrasound section.

(b)

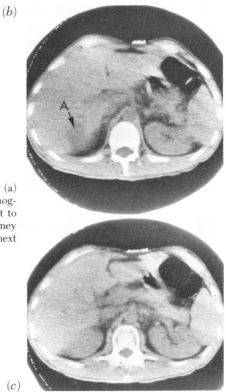

FIGURES 10B & C. The metastatic deposit (a) was missed on cross-section computed tomography because the metastasis was thought to represent the upper pole of the right kidney which appeared 13 mm caudad on the next section Figure 10c.

(c)

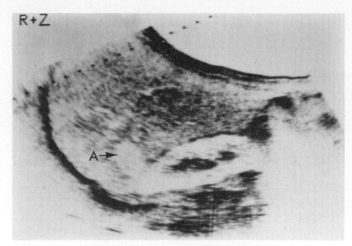

FIGURE 10D. A follow-up ultrasound examination 6 weeks later shows a 50% reduction in size of the lesion (a) in response to chemotherapy.

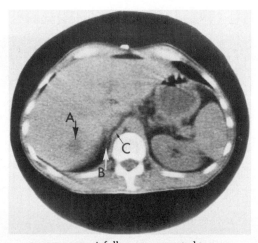

FIGURE 10E. A follow-up computed tomography examination 13 weeks after the first ultrasound and computed tomography exams shows the metastasis still present (a). It is small now and therefore easily placed within liver parenchyema. The right adrenal gland (b) is seen. A "bump" (c) on the right diaphragmatic crus represents a normal variant.

phrotoxic. In at least one instance at this institution these two drugs have apparently had synergistic nephrotoxic effects which resulted in acute renal failure within 24 hr of the administration of 100 cc 50% sodium diatrizoate intravenously.

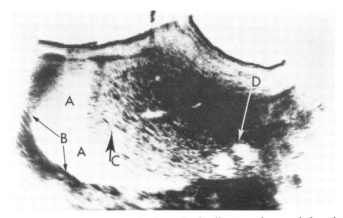

FIGURE 11. Ultrasound clearly places fluid collections above or below the diaphragm. In this testicular cancer patient the subdiaphragmatic abscess (a) is clearly located between the right diaphragm (b) and the liver (c). The tip of a hydronephrotic kidney (d) is also seen. While fluid can be detected on computed tomography, cross-section imaging can make it difficult to determine whether the fluid is above or below the diaphragm.

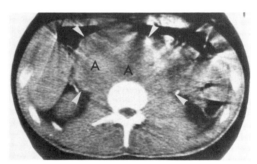

FIGURE 12A. Computed tomography shows a large mass (a), occupying the midabdomen in this patient.

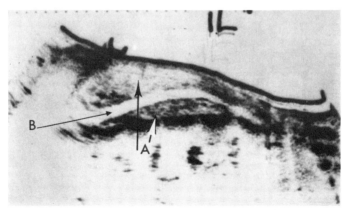

FIGURE 12B. Ultrasound scan not only shows the mass (a), but gives information about the location of the abdominal aorta (b), which is lifted ventrally and encased by the mass.

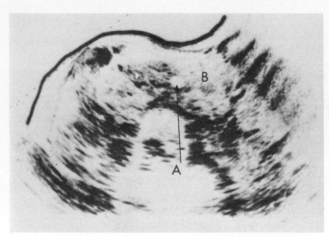

FIGURE 12C. A cross-section ultrasound shows the aorta (a), encased by the mass (b).

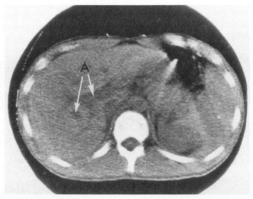

FIGURE 13. Branching portal veins (a) in the liver can simulate metastatic disease unless they are opacified by iodinated contrast media administered intravenously.

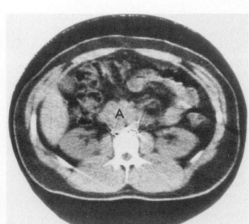

FIGURE 14A. Computed tomography done without orally administered contrast appears to show a mass (a), surrounding the great vessels.

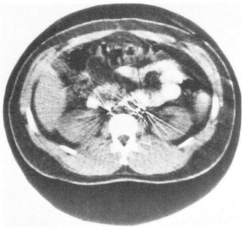

FIGURE 14B. After the administration of contrast media orally small bowel loops are opacified. A cut taken at the same level in 14a shows that the "mass" is really small bowel.

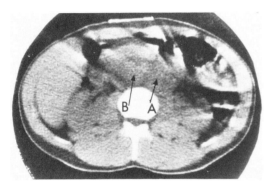

FIGURE 15A. Computed tomography shows classic periaortic (a) and pericaval (b) retroperitoneal lymphadenopathy from metastatic testicular cancer.

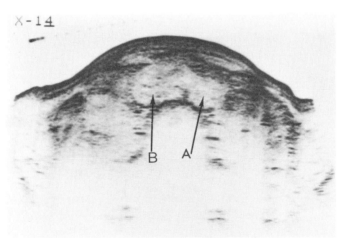

FIGURE 15B. Periaortic (a) and pericaval (b) adenopathy can also be seen with ultrasound in the same patient.

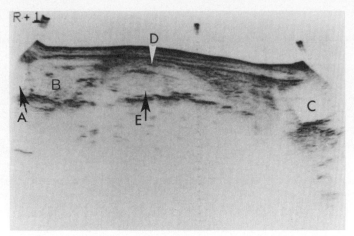

FIGURE 15C. A longitudinal ultrasound examination shows the heart (a), left lobe of the liver (b), and the urinary bladder (c). The aorta (d) is lifted ventrally, and the mass (e) is seen to lie almost entirely behind the vessel.

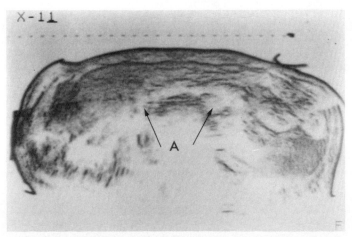

FIGURE 15D. A follow-up ultrasound examination at the same level as the initial computed tomography scan shows marked improvement in response to chemotherapy. Residual tumor (a) is located immediately ventral to each psoas muscle.

This directly contributed to the patient's death, even though he was being actively hydrated at the time of administration. For this reason we no longer give intravenous contrast material to patients receiving platinum chemotherapy. Fortunately testicular cancer does not often metastasize to the liver and ultrasound can accurately diagnose liver metastases and renal obstruction.[13]

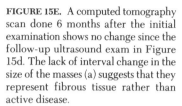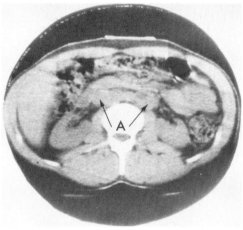

FIGURE 15E. A computed tomography scan done 6 months after the initial examination shows no change since the follow-up ultrasound exam in Figure 15d. The lack of interval change in the size of the masses (a) suggests that they represent fibrous tissue rather than active disease.

Small bowel loops may be confused with enlarged retroperitoneal lymph nodes unless they are opacified with iodinated contrast material administered orally (Fig. 14). Gastrograffin and Oral Hypaque are both suitable. The contrast should be diluted to a 3% solution to avoid artifact production from dense contrast in bowel loops in motion during the scan. Contrast should be administered far enough in advance of the scan to have time to fill the small bowel. Several doses at short time intervals may be necessary to opacify the entire small bowel. Routine use of oral contrast is essential when looking for enlarged lymph nodes.

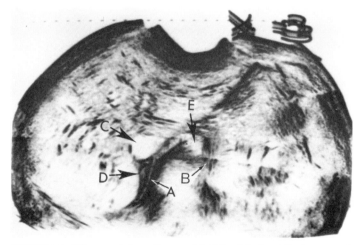

FIGURE 16A. Ultrasound shows the crus (a) of the right hemidiaphragm and the crus (b) of the left hemidiaphragm. The inferior vena cava (c) and the right adrenal gland (d) are not retrocrural. The aorta (e) is the only structure normally seen in the retrocrural space on ultrasound examination.

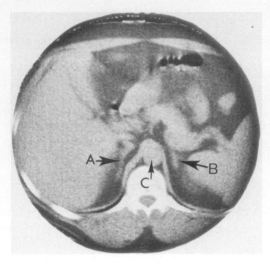

FIGURE 16B. Computed tomography in a different patient demonstrates the adrenal glands (a) and (b). Rarely computed tomography will show the azygous vein to the right of the aorta (c) in the retrocrural space.

Scan Findings

Massively enlarged lymph nodes in the periaortic and pericaval regions are easily diagnosed with ultrasound and computed tomography (Fig. 15). Enlarged lymph nodes in the retrocrural space high in the abdomen are also easily visualized (Figs. 16–18). Enlarged nodes in the pelvic region are less easily detected by both modalities because the great vessels no longer serve as landmarks and also because of confusion with the large ileal-psoas muscle bundles which lie immediately

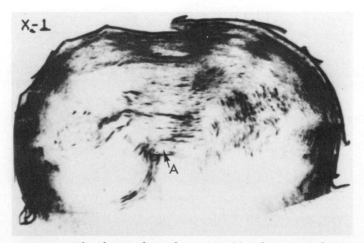

FIGURE 17A. This ultrasound scan shows a mass (a) in the retrocrural space representing lymphadenopathy from metastatic testicular carcinoma.

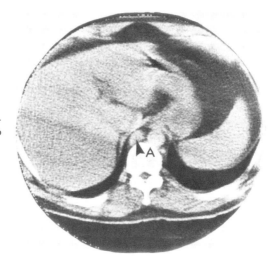

FIGURE 17B. A computed tomography slice at the same level also shows the metastatic disease(a).

subjacent to the lymphatic chains (Fig. 19). Pelvic disease is still readily detectable if a mass of any size is present (Fig. 20).

Reduction in the size of masses in response to chemotherapy is readily appreciated on both ultrasound and computed tomography scans (Fig. 21). A mass may shrink considerably but not completely disappear, or it may disappear entirely. In those cases where a mass shrinks but some residual mass remains, we have been unable to distinguish masses containing active neoplasm from those representing only residual fibrous tissue on a single scan.[14] Increase or decrease in size with time almost certainly indicates active disease (Fig. 22). Small residual masses may be surgically removed.

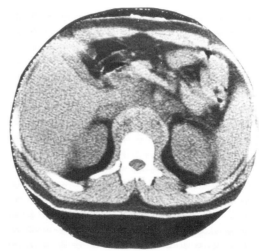

FIGURE 18. This patient exhibits massive, bilateral retrocrural disease.

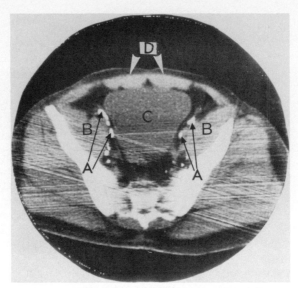

FIGURE 19. Computed tomography of the pelvis following lymphangiography shows normal opacified lymph nodes (a), immediately adjacent to the large ileopsoas muscle bundles (b). The urinary bladder (c) and rectus muscles (d) are also seen.

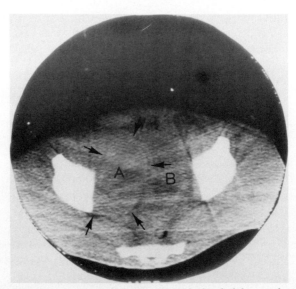

FIGURE 20. Computed tomography at the level of the acetabulum in a patient with no fat still shows a large pelvic mass (a), displacing the bladder (b).

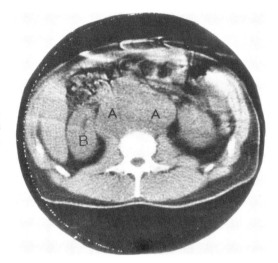

FIGURE 21A. Computed tomography initially shows a large mass (a), displacing the right kidney (b), laterally.

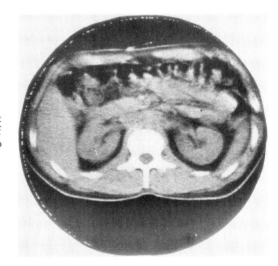

FIGURE 21B. A follow up scan at the same level after 4 months of chemotherapy has returned to normal.

Interval reduction in size is not the only indication of response to chemotherapy. In a number of cases a solid mass has become cystic on ultrasound, without any change in size (Fig. 23). Any cystic change on ultrasound indicates tumor necrosis, usually in response to chemotherapy. Confusion with lymphoceles should not be a problem as only one lymphocele was encountered in over 140 patients, and the diagnosis was readily established by needle aspiration (Fig. 24).

Change from high to low density on computed tomography indicates tumor necrosis in the same fashion as cystic changes on ultrasound. Caution must be exercised here because there are some very-low-density metastases on computed

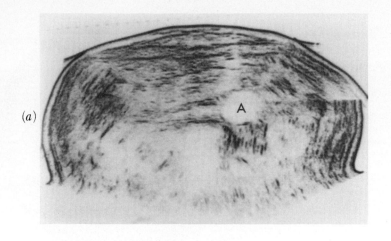

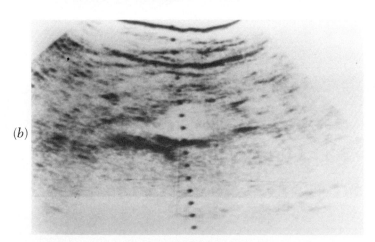

FIGURES 22A & B. Ultrasound shows an acoustically homogeneous abdominal mass (a), which does not change in size or texture on a follow up scan four months later (Fig. 22b). Normal alpha-fetoprotein and human chronic gonadotropin levels coupled with the ultrasound findings allowed this mass to be followed rather than resected.

tomography that are not cystic on ultrasound (Fig. 25). A good imaging end point indicating total tumor cell kill, other than complete lack of change over a long period of time, has not been found.

Computed tomography of the abdomen also has the advantage of displaying the lung bases. Frequently metastatic lesions are found in the lung bases which are not visible on chest radiographs or whole lung tomography (Fig. 26).

Computed tomography routinely demonstrates large masses in patients that have undergone lymphangiography. Quite frequently lymphangiographic

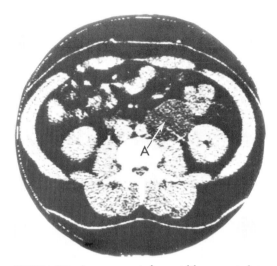

FIGURE 22C. A narrow window width computed tomography scan in the same patient demonstrates the low
density frequently associated with necrotic tumor (a).

contrast is not present in the largest and most abnormal nodes (Figs. 27–30).
Disease high in the abdomen, well seen on computed tomography, is frequently
devoid of lymphangiographic contrast. Of course lymphangiography cannot
provide information about the status of other intraabdominal organs. Ultrasound
and computed tomography may be repeated frequently to follow a patient, while
it is contraindicated to do repeated lymphangiograms in a short time period.

Accuracy

290 ultrasound examinations and 188 computed tomography examinations
were performed on 136 patients with prior orchiectomies for carcinoma of the
testicle. The examinations were reinterpreted by the authors and the results
compared with original reports and clinical, surgical, and pathologic findings.

Reinterpretation results agreed with the original report 83% of the time for
ultrasound and 87% of the time for computed tomography. Interobserver
agreement was 80% for ultrasound and 88% for computed tomography.

Thus computed tomography interpretation appears to be slightly more re-
producible than ultrasound interpretation from one observer to the next.[14]

Evaluation of the accuracy of computed tomography and ultrasound for detection of retroperitoneal lymphadenopathy was carried out. Ultrasound alone
had 7% false positives, 15% false negatives, 72% correct, and 7% equivocal.
Computed tomography had 7% false positives, 12% false negatives, 73% correct,
and 6% equivocal. There is no significant difference in the accuracy of ultrasound

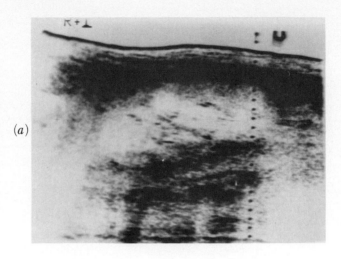

(a)

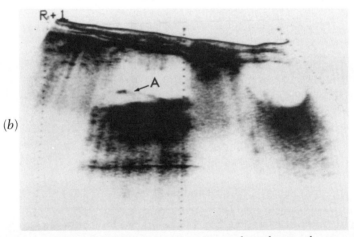

(b)

FIGURES 23A & B. Ultrasound best demonstrates response to chemotherapy when a mass changes from solid figure (a) to cystic figure (b). Only a thin membrane (a) remains in this large metastasis, which has otherwise become necrotic in response to chemotherapy.

compared to the accuracy of computed tomography for the detection of enlarged retroperitoneal lymph nodes. Overall accuracy rates in the study may be somewhat below those elsewhere in the literature because all patients were scanned in a prospective fashion and the scans interpreted as much as possible in spite of bowel gas artifacts on ultrasound and surgical clip artifacts on computed tomography. Also, early in the study oral contrast was not routinely used for computed tomography studies.

In another facet of study ultrasound and computed tomography exams done

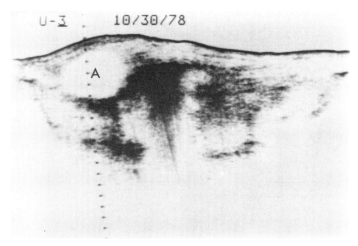

FIGURE 24. Lymphoceles are best evaluated by ultrasound. This lymphocele (a) shows the usual findings of being perfectly cystic with thin walls. Lymphoceles may be drained under ultrasound guidance if they are too deep or too small to be approached without guidance.

on the same patient within 1 week of one another were interpreted as if they represented a single examination, and a single overall diagnostic opinion was reached. In this situation interobserver agreement was 92%. Accuracy analysis showed 0% false positive, 14% false negative, 74% correct, and 12% equivocal. Equivocal exams were those where ultrasound and computed tomography seemed to disagree with each other. All false negatives were cases of minimal disease still intranodal in location. Of course, neither ultrasound nor computed tomography presently can image microscopic disease *in vivo*.

TABLE I
Accuracy of Lymphangiography Compared to Surgery

Author	Date	Number of patients	False positive	False negative	Correct positive	Correct negative	Equivocal
Seitzman	1964	21	2	6	7	6	0
Cook	1965	19	0	4	7	8	2
T. deRoo	1973	10	0	1	9	0	0
Safer	1975	35	4	3	8	18	0
Wallace	1970	67	1	8	17	41	0
Storm	1977	45	7	10	10	18	0
Kademian	1977	45	1	4	28	12	0
Fein	1969	50	0	10	20	20	0
Jonsson	1973	22	1	2	10	9	0
Maier	1972	69	3	6	42	6	0

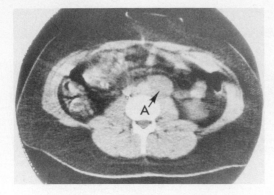

FIGURE 25A. Initial computed tomography examination in this patient shows periaortic metastatic disease (a).

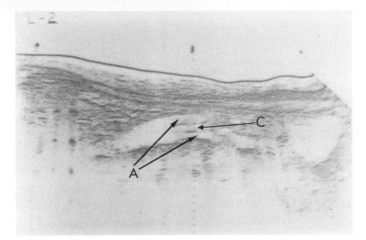

FIGURE 25B. A parasagittal ultrasound examination confirms the finding and shows the mass (a), surrounding the aorta (c).

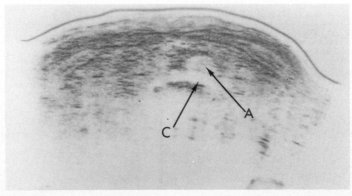

FIGURE 25C. Cross-sectional ultrasound imaging shows the mass (a) and is solid in relation to the "cystic" aorta (c).

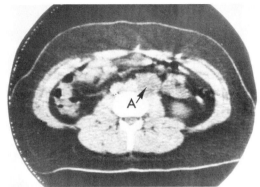

FIGURE 25D. Follow-up computed tomography after 2 months chemotherapy shows no significant change in the size of the mass (a). There is a suggestion that the mass is slightly more lucent.

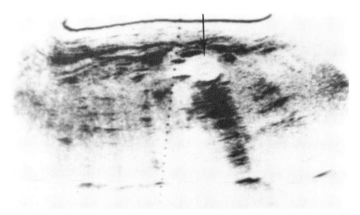

FIGURE 25E. A follow-up ultrasound exam on the same date as the computed tomography exam in Figure 25d demonstrates that the entire mass (arrow) has become cystic in response to chemotherapy. Such solid to cystic change indicates tumor necrosis in response to chemotherapy.

The above accuracy rates compare very favorably with the accuracy of lymphangiography. A review of the literature[15-24] (Table I) showed 5% false positive, 14% false negative, 80% correct, and 1% equivocal for lymphangiography. Ultrasound and computed tomography are noninvasive, can be repeated frequently, and provide more complete information about the extent of metastatic disease and its response to therapy. Lymphangiography is invasive, technically difficult, and cannot be repeated frequently.

Ultrasound can be used instead of intravenous pyelography for detecting renal obstruction. Ureteral deviation is a sign of gross disease that should be well seen on ultrasound and computed tomography scans.

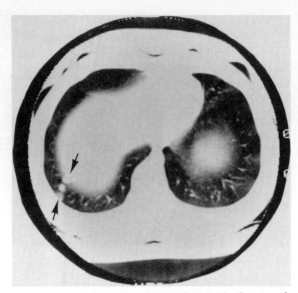

FIGURE 26. Computed tomography frequently detects pulmonary metastases in the costophrenic angles of the lung not visible on chest radiographs or whole lung tomography. This case shows three metastases (arrows) from testicular carcinoma in the right costophrenic angle. The lung bases should be examined routinely as part of the abdominal computed tomography exam in any patient with carcinoma of the testicle.

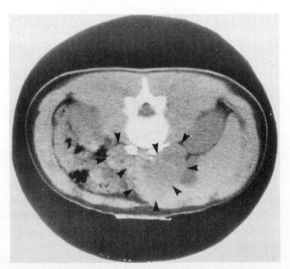

FIGURE 27. Computed tomography shows a large mass (arrows). Ethiodol from a lymphangiogram performed elsewhere is restricted to normal size retroperitoneal lymph nodes.

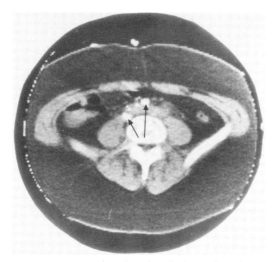

FIGURE 28A. Normal size lymph nodes (arrows) are shown opacified by Ethiodol near the bifurcation of the great vessels.

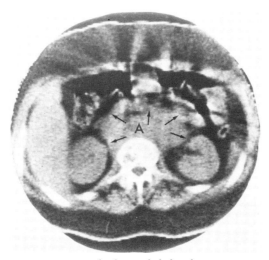

FIGURE 28B. A cut farther cephalad in the same patient shows a large mass (a) at the renal hilus level with no Ethiodol in it.

Summary

Testicular carcinoma patients should have an initial evaluation with both ultrasound and computed tomography, preferably on the same day. Both exami-

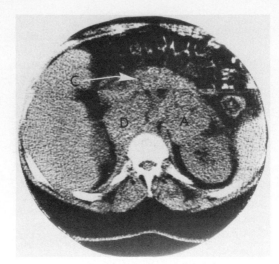

FIGURE 28C. A cut even farther cephalad demonstrates periaortic (a) and pericaval (d) lymph node masses behind the pancreas (c). Note the lack of Ethiodol in the masses in figures b & c. Lymphangiography has a good positive-negative accuracy rate, but it frequently greatly under-estimates the amount and extent of disease present, especially high in the abdomen.

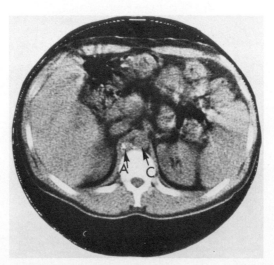

FIGURE 29. Rarely a lymphangiogram will show disease high in the abdomen. This patient had lymphangiography elsewhere prior to his computed tomography examination. Ethiodol is shown (a) in an enlarged retrocrural lymph node to the right of the aorta (c).

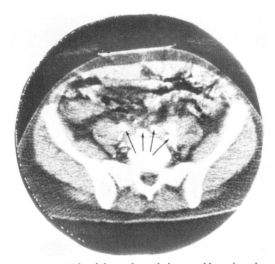

FIGURE 30. Ethiodol in enlarged abnormal lymph nodes (arrows) can aid in the interpretation of equivocal computed tomography scans, especially in the pelvic region. Ethiodol will mark lymph node location in the pelvis on computed tomography long after it has ceased to be useful for plain film follow-up of nodal architecture.

nations should be interpreted by the same radiologist, who should arrive at a single overall diagnostic opinion. When ultrasound and computed tomography findings seem contradictory, the results should be considered equivocal, and both exams should be repeated or lymphangiography may be performed. Another alternative is initial therapy based on chest x-ray findings and human chronic gonadotropin and alpha feto-protein values.[25–27]

Once metastatic disease is identified, it seems reasonable to follow it with ultrasound alone. Evaluation to substantiate the disease-free state and evaluation prior to retroperitoneal lymph node dissection should be done with both modalities.

The routine use of lymphangiography and intravenous pyelography is unnecessary in the testicular cancer patient population.

References

1. Einhorn, L., and Donohue, J.; Cis-Diamminedichloroplatinum, vinblastine, and bleomycin combination chemotherapy in disseminated testicular cancer. *Ann Intern Med* **87**(3): 293–298, 1977.

2. Gosink, B. B.: The inferior vena cava: mass effects. *Am J Roentgenol* **130**:533–536, 1978.

3. Tyrrel, C. J., Cosgrove, D. O., McCready, V. R., *et al.*: The role of ultrasound in the assessment and treatment of abdominal metastases from testicular tumors. *Clin Radiol* 28(5):475–481, 1977.

4. Tyrrell, C. J., Cosgrove, D. O., and McCready, V. R.: The assessment of abdominal lymph-nodes with ultrasound. *Br J Radiol* 49:732, 1976.

5. Kreel, L.: The EMI whole body scanner in the demonstration of lymph node enlargement. *Clin Radiol* 27(4):421–429, 1976.

6. Marshall, W. H., Jr., Breiman, R. S., Harell, G. S., *et al.*: Computed tomography of abdominal paraortic lymph node disease: preliminary observations with a 6 second scanner. *Am J Roentgenol* 128(5):759–764, 1977.

7. Brascho, D. J., Durant, J. R., and Green, L. E.: The accuracy of retroperitoneal ultrasonography in Hodgkin's disease and non-Hodgkin's lymphoma. *Radiology* 125(2):485–487, 1977.

8. Alcorn, F. S., Mategrano, V. C., Petasnick, J. P., *et al.*: Contributions of computed tomography in the staging and management of malignant lymphoma. *Radiology* 125(3): 717–723, 1977.

9. Jones, S. E., Tobias, D. A., and Waldman, R. S.: Computed tomographic scanning in patients with lymphoma. *Cancer* 41(2):480–486, 1978.

10. Redman, H. C., Glatstein, E., Castellino, R. A., and Federal, W. A.: Computed tomography as an adjunct in the staging of Hodgkin's disease and non-Hodgkin's lymphomas. *Radiology* 124(2):381–385, 1977.

11. Miller, R. E., Chernish, S. M., Brunelle, R. L., and Rosenak, B. D.: Double-blind radiographic study of dose response to intravenous glucagon for hypotonic duodenography. *Radiology* 127(1):55–59, 1978.

12. Von Holst, H., *et al.*: Titanium clips in neurosurgery for elimination of artifacts in computer tomography (A technical note). *Acta Neurochir (Wien)* 38(1–2):101–109, 1977.

13. Ellenberger, P. H., Scheible, W. F., Talner, L. A., and Leopold, F.: Sensitivity of grey scale ultrasound in detecting urinary tract obstruction. *Am J Roentgenol* 130:731–733, 1978.

14. Burney, B. T., and Klatte, E. C.: Ultrasound and computed tomography of the abdomen in the staging and management of testicular carcinoma. Abstract in Scientific Program, presented at 64th Scientific Assembly and Annual Meeting: The Radiological Society of North America, 1978.

15. Sweitzman, D. M., and Halaby, F. A.: Lymphangiography: An evaluation of its applications. *J Urol* 91:301–305, 1964.

16. Cook, F. E., Lawrence, D. D., Snith, J. R., and Gritti, E. J.: Testicular carcinoma and lymphangiography. *Radiology* 84:420–427, 1965.

17. de Roo, T., and van Minden, S. H.: Lymphographic findings in a series of 258 patients with tumors of the testes. *Lymphology* 6:97–100, June 1973.

18. Safer, M. L., Green, J. P., Crews, Q. E., and Hill, D. R.: Lymphangiographic accuracy in the staging of testicular tumors. *Cancer* 35(6):1603–1605, 1975.

19. Wallace, S., and Jing, B. S.: Lymphangiography: diagnosis of nodal metastases from testicular malignancies. *J Am Med Assoc* 213:94–96, 6 July 1970.

20. Storm, P. B., Kern, A., Loening, S. A., Brown, R. C., and Culp, D. A.: Evaluation of pedal lymphangiography in staging non-seminomatous testicular carcinoma. *J Urol* 118(6): 1002–1003, 1977.

21. Kademian, M., and Wirtanen, G.: Accuracy of bipedal lymphangiography in testicular tumors. *Urology* 9(2):218–220, 1977.

22. Fein, R. L., and Taber, D. O.: Foot lymphography in the testis tumor patient. *Cancer* 24:248–255, 1969.

23. Johsson, K., Ingemansson, S., and Ling, L.: Lymphography in patients with testicular tumours. *Br J Urol* **45**:548–554, 1973.

24. Maier, J. G., and Schamber, D. T.: The role of lymphangiography in the diagnosis and treatment of malignant testicular tumors. *Am J Roentgenol* **114**:482–491, 1972.

25. Grigor, K. M., Detre, S. I., Kohn, J., and Neville, A. M.: Serum alpha-foetoprotein levels in 153 male patients with germ cell tumours. *Br J Cancer* **35**(1):52–58, 1977.

26. Scardino, P. T., Cox, H. D., Waldmann, T. A., *et al.*: The value of serum tumor markers in the staging and prognosis of germ cell tumors of the testis. *J Urol* **118**(6):994–999, 1977.

27. Lange, P. H., McIntire, K. R., Waldmann, T. A., *et al.*: Alpha-fetoprotein and human chorionic gonadotropin in the management of testicular tumors. *J Urol* **118**(4):593–596, 1977.

6

The Management of Disseminated Testicular Cancer*

Lawrence H. Einhorn, M.D. and Stephen D. Williams, M.D.

Department of Medicine, Indiana University Medical Center and Veterans Administration Hospital, Indianapolis, Indiana 46202

ALTHOUGH TESTICULAR CANCER accounts for only 1% of all malignant tumors in males, it ranks first in incidence of cancer death in the 25–34-year-old age group.[1] Thus, cancer of the testis has a significant impact on the social, economic, and emotional status of this young population.

Testicular cancer usually presents as a scrotal mass first noticed by the patient himself. The healthy appearance of the patient belies the serious nature of this neoplasm. The diagnosis is established by a high inguinal orchiectomy, and subsequent staging workup is described below. Less commonly, germinal neoplasms may be extragonadal, with presentation in the retroperitoneum, mediastinum, or pineal, and with normal testes. Extragonadal germinal neoplasms are frequently more difficult to manage because of the large bulk of disease present at the time of diagnosis, and will be discussed separately in a later chapter.

* Supported in part by PHS Grant M01 RR00 750-06.

Histology and Staging

Histologically, testicular cancer is classified as shown in Table I. Although there are other pathological classifications, the Dixon-Moore one is the most widely used *clinical* classification. In the United States, the important distinction is whether the patient has a pure seminoma, as the management for seminomatous and nonseminomatous tumors markedly differs. Radiotherapy is the treatment of choice for pure seminoma, as this tumor is exquisitely radiosensitive, achieving a 90–95% cure rate in localized disease, and retroperitoneal node dissection is rarely indicated.[2] Radiotherapy for localized metastatic or recurrent seminoma has produced a 55% 5-year survival in one series.[3] The treatment of disseminated seminoma with chemotherapy will be discussed in a later chapter.

Although the proper therapy for most seminomas is orchiectomy plus radio-therapy, a word of caution should be interjected. Patients who have a "pure seminoma" diagnosed by orchiectomy should never have an elevated alpha-fetoprotein (AFP) level, because such patients have nonseminomatous elements present elsewhere. These patients should *not* be irradiated, but should be treated as nonseminomatous cancer.[4] There is very little argument concerning this statement, but there is considerably more controversy concerning the manage-ment of patients with pure seminoma and normal AFP but elevated beta-human chorionic gonadotropin (HCG). Generally speaking, it has been our policy to likewise treat such patients as "nonseminomatous" tumors, and to utilize retro-peritoneal lymphadenectomy rather than radiation therapy for clinical Stage I or II disease.

Testicular cancer is staged according to the extent of involvement (Table II). In the United States, the standard approach for nonseminomatous testicular cancer that is not Stage III is an ipsilateral or bilateral retroperitoneal lymphad-enectomy.[5] The staging workup commonly employed is shown in Table III. Obviously, the detection of pulmonary metastases is of crucial importance, as this would mitigate against a surgical approach. Routine PA and lateral chest x-rays can miss small pulmonary metastases that are visible with whole lung to-mograms. At Indiana University, we have not been impressed with the accuracy of lymphangiography or intravenous pyelography in testis tumors; thus, we presently evaluate the retroperitoneum with abdominal computerized tomog-

TABLE I.
Histology

Dixon-Moore	Histology
I	Pure seminoma
II	Embryonal, with or without seminoma
III	Teratoma
IV	Teratocarcinoma with embryonal or choriocarcinoma
V	Choriocarcinoma with embryonal carcinoma

TABLE II.

Stage

  I. Limited to testis alone
 II. Testis and retroperitoneal nodes
III. Supradiaphragmatic involvement

---

raphy and ultrasound, and do not employ the former studies. Radionucleotide studies of the liver, bone, or brain scans should be utilized in the staging workup only if clinically indicated. The value of serum alphafetoprotein (AFP) and human chorionic gonadotropin (HCG) measured by double antibody radioimmunoassays in staging, management, and follow-up of testicular germ cell tumors is well established.[6] Basically, the staging workup is performed to determine whether or not the patient has Stage III disease, and, thus, would be a candidate for chemotherapy instead of retroperitoneal lymphadenectomy. The remainder of this chapter will deal with the management of patients with Stage III disseminated testicular cancer. About 15–20% of patients with germinal testicular neoplasms present with Stage III disease; furthermore, about 10% of Stage I and 40%–50% of Stage II patients with nonseminomatous testicular cancer will recur as Stage III disease after primary surgical therapy.

Historical Perspectives

In 1960, Li and associates introduced the first major thrust of chemotherapy in advanced testicular cancer with the combination of actinomycin-D, chlorambucil, and methotrexate.[7] Subsequent studies confirmed a 50–70% response rate, which included 10–20% complete remissions.[8,9] During the past decade, several single agents have also been demonstrated to exhibit similar activity, namely vinblastine,[10] mithramycin,[11] and bleomycin.[12] The results of these and other early clinical trials is depicted in Table IV. The major significant achievements of these earlier studies was not only the demonstration that a complete remi_sion could be obtained in disseminated testicular cancer, but that approximately half of these complete remissions were permanent cures.[8–11]

TABLE III.

Staging Workup

History and Physical
Chest x-ray and whole lung tomograms
Beta subunit human chorionic gonadtropin
Alphafetoprotein
Bipedal lymphangiogram and/or abdominal CAT scan and ultrasound

---

TABLE IV.
Results with Early Chemotherapy Trials in Disseminated Testicular Cancer

Author	Treatment	Total number of patients	Complete remissions	Prolonged survivors[a]
Wyatt[13]	Methotrexate	10	4 (40%)	4
MacKenzie[9]	Actinomycin-D (alone or with chlorambucil ± methotrexate)	154	24 (16%)	13
Samuels[10]	Vinblastine	21	4 (1)	2
Kennedy[11]	Mithramycin	23	5 (22%)	5
Mendelson[14]	Cyclophosphamide + vincristine + methotrexate + fluorouracil (COMF)	17	5 (2)	1

[a] Refers to those patients remaining alive and disease-free at the time of publication.

Furthermore, most of those patients who relapsed did so within 1 year of achieving complete remission, with a smaller percentage of relapses occurring during the second year. Relapses occurring after 2 years of a chemotherapy-induced complete remission have been anecdotal. Thus, if a patient with Stage III nonseminomatous testicular cancer has been continuously disease-free for 2 years, he is probably cured of of his malignancy.

Although it is encouraging that approximately 50% of these complete remissions were apparent cures, it is expected that modern combination chemotherapy today will have a considerably lower relapse rate for those patients achieving complete remission because of more effective remission induction therapy with platinum combination chemotherapy (*vide infra*) and because of the increased accuracy in defining complete remission today (radioimmunoassay beta-HCG, AFP, whole lung tomograms, abdominal CAT scan, abdominal ultrasound).

Another point of particular interest in these earlier studies was the durability of complete remission with mithramycin despite the absence of maintenance therapy.[11] Kennedy utilized mithramycin for 6 months, and then stopped all therapy. It is quite possible that maintenance therapy is unnecessary in disseminated testicular cancer. Similar situations exist in other chemosensitive tumors such as Hodgkin's disease where maintenance therapy is apparently unnecessary.[15]

Vinblastine + Bleomycin

Combination chemotherapy with vinblastine + bleomycin in disseminated testicular cancer was pioneered by Samuels, and represented a major advance in that disease.[16-18] This two-drug regimen is an apparently synergistic regimen, producing higher complete remission rates than would be predicted by the single agent data. A possible explanation for this synergism is that bleomycin, *in vitro*, is most effective in killing Chinese hamster ovary cells in mitosis,[19] and vinblastine produces an arrest in the mitotic phase of the cell cycle.

Initial studies with vinblastine + bleomycin (VB-I) were started by Samuels in 1970, using dosages of 0.4–0.6 mg/kg of vinblastine plus bleomycin 15 mg/M² twice weekly.[17] There were 17 of 51 (33%) complete remissions with VB-I in disseminated nonseminomatous testicular cancer with a relapse rate of 23%.

In 1973, bleomycin therapy was switched from intermittent therapy to continuous infusion (VB-III) (30 units in 1000 cc of 5% glucose and water over a 24-hr period for 5 consecutive days starting on day 2).[16] Vinblastine was given in a total dose of 0.4 mg/kg split into two fractions on days 1 and 2, but no less than 30 mg as the initial loading dosage.[17] Therapy was repeated every 28–35 days as toxicity permitted. The rationale for continuous infusion bleomycin was based upon the data that the half-life is short (less than 2 hr) and tissue inactivation is rapid, and the drug is a cell-cycle specific drug acting at the G_2-M interphase.[16] Recently updated data for VB-III indicated a 53% complete remission rate (47/89 patients); relapse data was not available.[18]

The toxicity of these vinblastine + bleomycin programs have been well described in previous publications.[16,17] Bacteriologically proven sepsis was seen in 13% of these patients and was responsible for four drug-related deaths.[17] Bleomycin pulmonary fibrosis was seen in 7% of these patients, and half of the patients developing this complication died from pulmonary fibrosis.[17] However, there was no drug-induced mortality in any patient in complete remission.[17]

Although many groups continue to utilize continuous infusion bleomycin in testicular cancer and other malignancies, there is no firm data demonstrating its superiority over the more easily administered intermittent bleomycin. Table V compares VB-I, which was employed from 1970–1973, to VB-III which has been used since 1973. Although the complete remission rate appears higher for VB-III compared to the historical control VB-I, this possible superiority was only applicable for embryonal carcinoma (Table V).[17] It is thus unlikely that there would be a therapeutic advantage to using continuous infusion bleomycin in platinum + vinblastine + bleomycin combination chemotherapy because of the exceptionally high complete remission rate with this three-drug regimen.

TABLE V.
Continuous vs. Intermittent Bleomycin

	VB I			VB III		
	Total	CR (%)	PR (%)	Total	CR (%)	PR (%)
Embryonal	26	7 (26%)	13 (50%)	36	21 (58%)	13 (36%)
Teratocarcinoma	24	10 (44%)	5 (21%)	21	7 (33%)	0 (24%)
Choriocarcinoma	1	0	1	4	1 (25%)	0
Totals	51	17 (33%)	19 (37%)	61	29 (48%)	21 (34%)

Vinblastine + bleomycin represented a major advance in the early 1970's in the treatment of disseminated testicular cancer. Another major advance was the discovery of the activity of cis-diamminedichloroplatinum in germinal neoplasms. Cis-diamminedichloroplatinum is one of a group of coordination compounds of platinum identified by Rosenberg, VanCamp, and Krigas that strongly inhibits bacterial replication.[20] This agent has significant activity in refractory advanced testicular cancer and is ideal for combination chemotherapy because of its relative lack of myelosuppression.[21] It is our feeling that platinum is the single most active agent in testicular cancer, and should be an integral part of any combination chemotherapy program for disseminated testicular cancer.

VAB Programs—Memorial

The Memorial group evaluated combination chemotherapy with vinblastine + actinomycin-D + bleomycin (VAB-I) from June 1972 to April 1974.[22] This treatment regimen produced only 14% complete and 22% partial remissions in 71 evaluable patients.[23] Although the dosages and method of administration were markedly different from Samuels' vinblastine + bleomycin program, the rather low complete remission rate with VAB-I raises serious questions as to the role (if any) of actinomycin-D in modern day remission induction chemotherapy in testicular cancer.

VAB-II incorporated cis-diamminedichloroplatinum and continuous infusion bleomycin into the VAB protocol.[24,25] This protocol was utilized from June 1974 to January 1976 and produced a 50% complete and 34% partial remission rate in 50 evaluable patients.[25] An additional two patients were rendered disease-free by surgical resection of residual disease after a chemotherapy induced partial remission. There was a 60% complete and 36% partial response rate in previously untreated patients. The induction phase consisted of vinblastine 0.06 mg/kg and actinomycin-D 0.02 mg/kg on day 1. Bleomycin 0.5 mg/kg was given by continuous infusion for 7 days, and platinum was given in a dosage of 1 mg/kg on day 8. A weekly maintenance of vinblastine and bleomycin with actinomycin-D and platinum on a rotating schedule was given followed by vinblastine, actinomycin-D, and chlorambucil every 3–4 weeks. The induction course (vinblastine + actinomycin-D + bleomycin + platinum) was repeated 4 months after the start of therapy. Following this reinduction, maintenance was changed to vinblastine 0.1 mg/kg and actinomycin-D 0.025 mg/kg every 3 weeks and chlorambucil 0.1 mg/kg p.o. daily for a total of 2–3 years in the absence of relapse. There was one drug-related death in this series, and seven instances of allergic reactions to platinum. At the time of publication,[25] only 15 of 50 patients remain alive (30%) and only 12 (24%) are presently disease-free from 19 to 35 months following start of therapy. These results are markedly inferior to those achieved at Indiana University with platinum + vinblastine + bleomycin during a similar time period.

VAB III

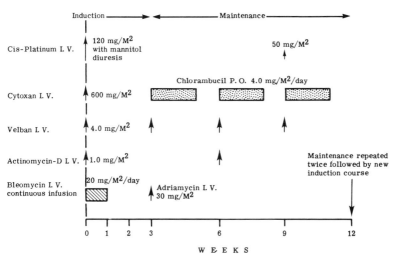

FIGURE 1. VAB III.

The Memorial group next evaluated a rather complicated regimen (VAB-III) shown in Fig. 1. Eighty patients were treated from 7/75 through 9/76 with a 63% complete and 35% partial remission rate.[23] With follow-up of 17–31 months, 44% of the VAB-III patients remain free of disease.[26]

Since September 1976, the Memorial group has been using VAB-IV using the same drugs and doses of VAB-III but with slight scheduling modifications and with similar therapeutic results to VAB-III.[23] The preliminary analysis of VAB-IV reveal 24–48 patients (50%) to be free of disease with a follow-up considerably shorter than for VAB-III.[26]

Platinum + Vinblastine + Bleomycin (PVB)—Indiana

In August 1974, we began a study using platinum + vinblastine + bleomycin in disseminated testicular cancer. It was our impression at that time that the best therapeutic results were achieved with vinblastine + bleomycin and that platinum, a highly active and relatively nonmyelosuppressive drug, was a logical candidate for addition to vinblastine + bleomycin.

Fifty patients with germ-cell tumors of the testis were entered from August 1974 through September 1976.[27] Three patients died within 2 weeks of initiation of chemotherapy and were considered inevaluable. The therapy regimen is depicted in Table VI. Platinum was dissolved in 50 cc sterile water and given as a 15-min infusion. Most patients received three courses of platinum; however, if

TABLE VI.

Platinum + Vinblastine + Bleomycin

Platinum 20 mg/M² IV × 5 days every 3 weeks (3–4 courses)	remission induction
Vinblastine 0.2 mg./kg. IV × 2 every 3 weeks (4 courses)	therapy
Bleomycin 30 units IV push weekly × 12	maintenance therapy
Vinblastine 0.3 mg/kg monthly × 21	

a complete remission was not achieved after 3 courses, a fourth course was administered. Vinblastine was given 6 hr prior to bleomycin in an attempt to synchronize tumor cells for maximal destruction by bleomycin. However, this kinetic scheduling is no longer felt to be necessary, and we now give vinblastine and bleomycin simultaneously. After completion of the 12 weeks of remission induction, maintenance therapy was given with vinblastine 0.3 mg/kg every 4 weeks for a total of 2 years of chemotherapy. Initially, bacillus Calmette-Guerin (BCG) immunotherapy was given if complete remission was achieved in an attempt to augment host cell mediated immunity and prolong the duration of complete remission. However, we have recently questioned the value of adding BCG to such patients, and in the past 2 years, we have not employed any form of immunotherapy. Since our relapse rate remains at a very low level despite cessation of BCG, it appears unlikely BCG contributed any therapeutic advantage.

The primary goal was to increase the complete remission rate and potential cure rate. Partial remission was not considered a worthwhile goal unless the patient was left with localized disease that could be surgically removed.

Thirty-three of 47 evaluable patients (70%) achieved complete remission (defined as a complete disappearance of all clinical, radiographic, and biochemical evidence of disease, including normal whole lung tomograms, serum beta-HCG, and AFP). The remaining 14 patients achieved partial remission (greater than 50% decrease of measurable disease). Furthermore, five of these 14 patients were rendered disease-free following surgical removal of residual localized disease after significant reduction of tumor volume with chemotherapy. The therapeutic results are outlined in Table VII.

These patients now have been followed for 28–52 months, and they are all off chemotherapy. The survival curve is shown in Figure 2. Four patients died in complete remission in the early part of this study. Two of these deaths were due to gram-negative sepsis, one from bleomycin-induced pulmonary fibrosis, and one from multiple small bowel fistulae and obstruction secondary to previous surgery. One of the septicemia deaths was from Klebsiella pneumonia in a chronic alcoholic who had no evidence of granulocytopenia during this fatal pneumonia. Thusly, this regimen was directly responsible for two drug-related fatalities. However, an additional 78 patients (*vide infra*) have been treated with platinum

TABLE VII.

Results with Platinum + Vinblastine + Bleomycin

Evaluable patients	47
Complete remission	33 (70%)
Partial remission	14 (30%)
Disease-free after surgery	5 (11%)
Number alive	32 (68%)
Number continuously NED	26 (55%)
Number presently NED	28 (60%)

+ vinblastine + bleomycin (+ adriamycin) and there were no drug-induced mortalities in this series of patient.

Only six of these 33 complete remissions have relapsed. Five of these relapses occurred within 9 months of initiation of complete remission and the sixth relapse

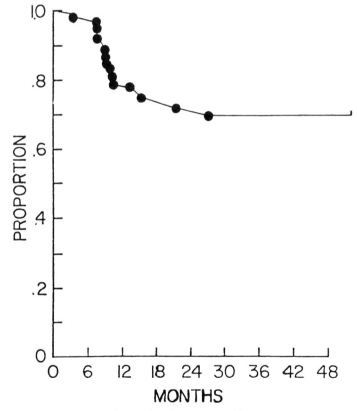

FIGURE 2. Survival curve for platinum + vinblastine + bleomycin.

occurred at 17 months. Since all of these patients have been followed for a minimum of 28 months, it is highly probable that the rest of these patients are cured of their malignancy, as "late" relapses are uncommon even with less effective chemotherapy.[7-11] Three of these patients achieved a brief second complete remission with platinum + adriamycin + bleomycin + vincristine. Interestingly, two of these patients are presently in a prolonged third complete remission with platinum + VP-16, an epipodophyllotoxin derivative. Our experience with VP-16 in testicular cancer will be described in a subsequent chapter.

As previously mentioned, five of the 14 partial remissions were rendered free of disease by surgical removal of residual localized disease. It has been our treatment policy to do surgery on these patients only if they have persistent localized disease following four courses of platinum + vinblastine + bleomycin. Usually, this clinical situation occurs in patients with Stage III disease who exhibit complete disappearance of pulmonary metastases (confirmed by whole lung tomograms) but still have persistent abdominal disease (as per physical examination, abdominal ultrasound, or abdominal CAT scan). It should be noted that those patients who present *de novo* with Stage III disease and achieve complete remission are *not* subjected to a laparotomy (i.e., only those patients with clinical or radiographic evidence of residual abdomen disease). We do not feel such patients need a laparotomy and retroperitoneal node dissection merely because they never had a node dissection originally, but rather reserve laparotomy only if there is evidence of persistent abdominal disease. Furthermore, we do not do laparotomies on such patients achieving chemotherapeutic partial remissions if they have evidence of remaining pulmonary metastases. Using this criteria for laparotomy, about one-third of these patients will have persistent carcinoma, one-third will have transformed to benign mature teratoma, and one-third will have fibrous tissue only. These figures apply to all patients seen at Indiana University with disseminated testicular cancer.

The transformation of malignant embryonal carcinoma to benign mature teratoma with aggressive chemotherapy has previously been reported.[28,29] The malignant potential of these mature teratomas is unknown. Patients who had complete surgical removal of persistent carcinoma fared poorly compared to patients having only teratoma or fibrous tissue in the surgical specimen. All the patients in the latter two categories are presently disease-free, whereas only five of nine patients with carcinoma are presently free of disease. Other authors have also reported excellent results when the surgical specimen reveals conversion to mature teratoma after chemotherapy[30] and poor results when persistent carcinoma is found, even though it has been completely removed.[31] Obviously, such patients are at high risk for relapse, and it is our impression that those patients who have residual carcinoma in their surgical specimens (following a chemotherapy-induced partial remission) should be treated aggressively with an additional two to three courses of platinum + vinblastine + bleomycin postoperatively.

We have also performed thoracotomy on selected patients who achieved only

TABLE VIII.

Histology and Response

Histology	No. of patients	CR %
Pure seminoma	4	50%
Embryonal (± seminoma)	25	84%
Teratoma	2	50%
Teratocarcinoma	9	44%
Choriocarcinoma	5	60%
Yolk sac	2	100%

a partial remission with chemotherapy. These patients had no evidence of abdominal disease, and had solitary pulmonary nodules remaining after significant cytoreduction with chemotherapy. Although the numbers are smaller, the patterns are very similar to the above mentioned laparotomy results.

The relationship of histology to response is shown in Table VIII. Excellent complete remission rates were seen in all cell types, although there was a suggestion of a higher complete remission rate in embryonal carcinoma. Because of our continuted high complete remission rate in embryonal carcinoma, we have not been inclined to switch our method of administration of bleomycin from intermittent weekly to continuous infusion, as the latter method was shown to have a potential advantage in Samuels data only for embryonal carcinoma.[17]

The most important determinant for achieving complete remission is extent of metastatic disease (Table IX). Advanced pulmonary disease was defined as pulmonary metastases greater than 2 cm in diameter, and advanced abdominal disease was present if there was a palpable abdominal mass or the presence of hepatic metastases. Nineteen of 22 patients with minimal disease (groups A, C, and E, in Table IX) achieved complete remission, and one patient was rendered free of disease after surgical removal of a benign mature teratoma at thoracotomy. The only patients with minimal metastatic disease failing to achieve complete remission all had prior chemotherapy and/or radiotherapy.

TABLE IX.

Extent of Disease and Response

	No. of patients	CR %
A. Minimal pulmonary disease	10	80%
B. Advanced pulmonary disease	9	67%
C. Minimal abdominal and pulmonary disease	9	88%
D. Advanced abdominal disease	16	50%
E. Elevated HCG alone	3	100%

Radioimmunoassay AFP was elevated in 40% of the patients and HCG in 75%. Only three patients failed to have either marker elevated. Those patients achieving complete remission usually have at least a one log reduction in their marker(s) with each course of platinum combination chemotherapy.

The relationship of prior therapy to complete remission is shown in Table X. There was a lower complete remission rate in patients with prior radiotherapy, and these patients had considerably more prolonged and severe hematological and gastrointestinal toxicity. We routinely lower the dosage of vinblastine 25% if a patient has had prior radiotherapy.

Although partial remission is not a worthwhile goal, it is noteworthy that three of these partial remissions remain in their original partial remission with bilateral pulmonary metastases for 2+ to $3\frac{1}{2}$+ years. These prolonged partial remissions are presumably further examples of histologic conversion to a more mature and benign form (teratoma), and the ultimate fate of these three patients remains to be determined.

Toxicity could be best described by separating this three-drug combination into its individual components:

Cis-platinum caused moderate to severe nausea and vomiting in all patients during each 5-day course. During the first year of this study, intravenous hydration was only employed for very severe nausea and vomiting. Although only three of these earlier patients had significant azotemia (blood urea nitrogen greater than 50 mg% and/or serum creatinine greater than 3.0 mg%), many of these earlier patients now have a 25–50% reduction from their baseline creatinine clearance and have serum creatinines of 1.5–2.0 mg%.[32] None of these patients show progressive nephrotoxicity or azotemic symptomatology, and the long-term effects of cis-platinum on renal function are still being studied. In the past 24 months, we have been employing vigorous intravenous hydration on all patients during each course of cis-platinum utilizing 100 cc/hr of normal saline for 12 hr prior to administration of chemotherapy (prehydration) and then continuous saline hydration during all 5 days of cis-platinum administration. Since we have been utilizing this form of intravenous hydration, we have only rarely encountered any of the above biochemical manifestations of platinum nephrotoxicity.

Table X.
Prior Therapy and Response

	No. of Pts.	CR %
Surgery alone	21	76%
Surgery + chemoprophylaxis	9	88%
Surgery + chemotherapy (for metastatic disease)	10	70%
Surgery + radiotherapy	3	33%
Surgery + chemotherapy radiotherapy	4	25%

In addition to preventing biochemical azotemia with saline hydration, we have also prevented anatomical abnormalities as demonstrated by light and electron microscopy of renal biopsy specimens performed during laparotomy for excision of residual abdominal disease. The sophisticated studies of Stark and Howell also showed a lack of nephrotoxicity with this chemotherapy regimen and saline hydration.[33] We have not employed mannitol diuresis in any of our patients. Although occasional patients had a decrease in high-frequency hearing, there were no observed clinical audiological abnormalities. Mild hyperuricemia, hypokalemia, hypocalcemia, and hypomagnesemia were occasionally seen, but was not a clinical problem.

Bleomycin produced fever, chills, and cutaneous striae in all patients, but these were not a clinical problem and did not require alteration of the bleomycin dosages. All patients had significant alopecia and most had weight loss (from cis-platinum and bleomycin) during the 12 weeks of bleomycin. The average weight loss was 20 pounds. No patient required intravenous hyperalimentation, and all patients completely regained their weight after the completion of bleomycin. There was one death from bleomycin pulmonary fibrosis; there were no other cases of clinically significant pulmonary fibrosis.

Vinblastine produced myalgia in half of the patients. Although this was occasionally severe enough to require narcotic analgesics during the first 12 weeks of therapy, it was only rarely a significant clinical problem during maintenance therapy with the lower dosage (0.3 mg/kg) of vinblastine. However, some patients still had severe myalgias even with the lowered dosage of vinblastine, and these patients usually had their dosage lowered to 0.2 mg/kg once a month. Anemia and thrombocytopenia were observed in several patients, but no patient had thrombocytopenic bleeding or required platelet transfusions. Only four patients experienced thrombocytopenia below 100,000, and these were all in patients who had prior radiotherapy. Anemia was more of a problem, especially in patients who had had prior radiotherapy. Packed red blood cell transfusions were required periodically on four patients during the first several months of therapy, and all four of these patients had received prior radiotherapy. Leukopenia also was more severe and prolonged in patients with prior irradiation and they were started on a lowered dosage of vinblastine (0.15 mg/kg for 2 consecutive days). The most serious side effect, which was seen in all patients, was severe leukopenia. The nadir of the white blood count usually was 1000 between days 7 and 14. Eighteen patients required hospitalization for presumed sepsis with granulocytopenic fever and were cultured and started on antibiotic coverage with broad-spectrum antibiotics. Seven of these patients had documented Gram-negative sepsis, and one of these patient died of sepsis.

Despite the aforementioned significant toxicity, this occurred primarily during the 12 weeks of remission induction therapy. Maintenance therapy with vinblastine was well tolerated, and all patients regained their hair growth and weight during this period. No patient required hospitalization for complications of therapy during vinblastine maintenance.

TABLE XI.
Clinical Data of Patients

Patient No.	Tumor type	Prior[a,b] therapy	Extent of disease	Response	Duration (months)	Survival (months)
1	Embryonal	1) RND + radiotherapy 2) VB 3) Actinomycin-D + cyclophosphamide + vincristine	1) massive bilat. pulmonary metastases	partial	7	10
2	Choriocarcinoma—primary mediastinal	VB	1) bilat. cervical nodes 2) large mediastinal mass 3) hepatic	partial	3	5
3	Teratocarcinoma	VB	1) peritracheal mass 2) retroperitoneal nodes	partial	5	11
4	Embryonal	1) Actinomycin-D 2) Mithramycin 3) Bleo-COMF 4) VB	1) cervical nodes 2) massive bilat. pulmonary metastases	partial	5	9
5	Embryonal—primary mediastinal	1) radiotherapy 2) VB	1) large mediastinal mass	partial	3	4
6	Teratocarcinoma	1) Actinomycin-D + Cytoxan 2) radiotherapy	1) massive bilat. pulm. metastases	partial	5	7

3) VB

7	Teratocarcinoma	1) RND + radiotherapy 2) VB 3) Actinomycin-D 4) Mithramycin	1) massive bilat. pulmonary metastases	partial	4	6
8	Teratocarcinoma	1) RND + radiotherapy 2) Actinomycin-D 3) VB	1) massive pulmonary metastases	complete	13	26
9	Teratocarcinoma	VB	1) retroperitoneal nodes 2) massive bilat. pulmonary metastases	partial	7	13
10	Teratocarcinoma	1) RND + radiotherapy 2) VB	1) cervical nodes 2) massive bilat. pulmonary metastases	partial	7	18+

[a] RND = retroperitoneal node dissection.
[b] VB = vinblastine + bleomycin.

The Southwest Oncology Group has also studied combination chemotherapy with platinum + vinblastine + bleomycin using a similar dosage schedule.[34] Fifty-seven evaluable patients were treated, and there were 32 complete remissions (56%) and 17 partial remissions (30%). It is noteworthy that this study employed a lower dosage of vinblastine (12 mg/M^2 every 4 weeks), and there were no toxic deaths. Numerous other institutions and cooperative groups also have used platinum + vinblastine + bleomycin with similar excellent results.

Platinum + Adriamycin

From 1974 to 1977, we have treated 10 patients with disseminated testicular cancer who failed to respond to vinblastine + bleomycin as employed at other institutions. These results were previously published.[35] Since these patients were refractory to adequate dosages of vinblastine plus bleomycin (usually VB III as described previously by Samuels), they were clearly not candidates for platinum, vinblastine, and bleomycin as that would be analogous to using single agent platinum. Adriamycin has activity as a single agent in testicular cancer,[36] although its exact role in this era of combination chemotherapy is difficult to ascertain. In addition, adriamycin is apparently synergistic with platinum,[37] and thus this two drug combination was tested in this refractory patient population.

Table XI summarizes the pertinent clinical data. None of these patients achieved complete remission on prior therapy. All patients had advanced pulmonary disease (pulmonary metastases greater then 2 cm in diameter), and three patients also had advanced abdominal disease (palpable abdominal mass or hepatic metastases).

Platinum was given in our usual dosage of 20 mg/M^2 for 5 consecutive days every 3 weeks. Two patients received three courses, six had four courses, and one patient had five and seven courses each of platinum. Adriamycin was given in a dosage of 60 mg/M^2 IV on the first day of platinum therapy every 3 weeks. The adriamycin dosage was reduced 20% in those patients who had prior radiotherapy. Maintenance therapy with adriamycin alone was given after completion of platinum until a total dosage of 550 mg/M^2 was reached. Only one patient (no. 10) received maintenance therapy with platinum (75 mg/M^2 once a month) plus adriamycin.

All 10 patients responded objectively to combination chemotherapy with cis-diamminedichloroplatinum plus adriamycin. However, only one patient achieved a complete remission. This patient relapsed after completion of maintenance adriamycin, and a brief second complete remission with platinum alone was achieved. Further attempts at remission induction were not successful, and he died of his neoplasm 26 months after initiation of platinum + adriamycin.

The median duration of remission was 5 months and the median survival was 9½ months. This was a very poor risk patient population, as all patients had massive pulmonary metastases, all had failed to respond to vinblastine plus bleomycin chemotherapy, five patients were previously refractory to at least one

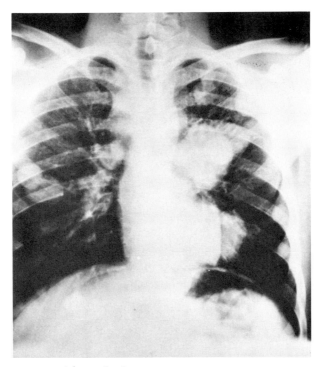

FIGURE 3. Advanced pulmonary metastases in patient 1.

other chemotherapy regimen, six patients had prior radiotherapy, and six patients had elevated alpha-fetoprotein levels. The far-advanced stage of this patient population is further demonstrated by the fact that five patients died within 2 months of their relapse on maintenance adriamycin.

Cis-diamminedichloroplatinum therapy was stopped because of stabilization of antineoplastic response with no further regression. Only one patient (no. 4) progressed while still on platinum. This patient received seven courses of platinum plus adriamycin with further regression with each course of therapy. However, when he was admitted for evaluation of an eighth course, he exhibited progressive pulmonary metastases.

Most relapses occurred in the areas of original disease; however, three patients relapsed in the central nervous system as a new anatomical site of disease while they were developing progressive pulmonary metastases.

Case Reports

Patient 1 was a 21-year-old male with embryonal testicular cancer treated initially with orchiectomy and postoperative radiotherapy. Several months after

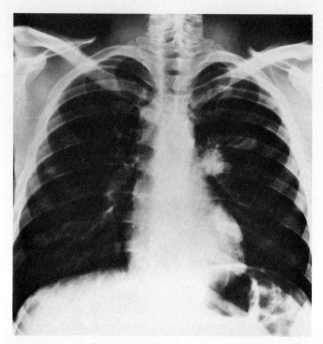

FIGURE 4. Marked regression after one course of platinum + adriamycin.

completion of irradiation, he developed bilateral pulmonary metastases and was treated with vinblastine + continuous infusion bleomycin without objective response. He then received combination chemotherapy with vincristine + actinomycin-D + cyclophosphamide with further progression, and he was subsequently referred to Indiana University. At the time of admission here, he was symptomatic with cough, shortness of breath, and dyspnea on exertion. He had lost 50 pounds in the preceding 6 months. Chest x-ray revealed massive bilateral pulmonary metastases (Fig. 3). Serum lactic dehydrogenase (LDH) was 482, beta subunit human chorionic gonadotrophin (B-HCG) was 4860, and alpha-fetoprotein (AFP) was 2100.

The patient was started on combination chemotherapy with cis-diamminedichloroplatinum 20 mg/M^2 for 5 consecutive days plus adriamycin 48 mg/M^2. Three weeks later, he returned for his second course of therapy, asymptomatic, and had gained 17 pounds. His chest x-ray after just one course of platinum plus adriamycin showed a marked regression in the bilateral pulmonary metastases (Fig. 4). He received a total of four courses of platinum + adriamycin, at which time his B-HCG, AFP, and LDH were all normal. However, his chest x-ray revealed persistent, stable small pulmonary metastases. He con-

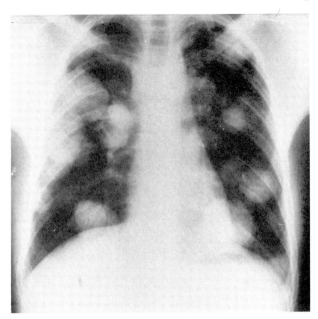

FIGURE 5. Massive pulmonary metastases in patient 7.

tinued maintenance chemotherapy with adriamycin 48 mg/M^2 once a month. However, 8 months after initiation of chemotherapy, he developed progressive pulmonary and retroperitoneal metastases, and his B-HCG again started to rise.

Shortly thereafter, he developed brain metastases, and, despite chemotherapy with mithramycin, he died 6 weeks after relapse. He had an excellent quality remission, remaining asymptomatic and gaining 30 pounds, and had a 10-month survival from initiation of platinum plus adriamycin chemotherapy.

Patient 7 was a 23-year-old male who underwent orchiectomy, retroperitoneal node dissection, and postoperative irradiation for teratocarcinoma. He subsequently developed pulmonary metastases, and he failed to respond to vinblastine plus continuous infusion bleomycin. He later developed further progression with both actinomycin-D and mithramycin before his referral to Indiana University. At the time of admission, he had a Karnofsky performance status of 50 with severe shortness of breath and dyspnea on exertion. Chest x-ray revealed massive pulmonary metastases (Fig. 5). He was started on adriamycin 48 mg/M^2 plus cis-diamminedichloroplatinum 20 mg/M^2 × 5 days. Three weeks later, he was readmitted for his second course of therapy, asymptomatic, and with a dramatic regression in the size and number of pulmonary metastases (Fig. 6). He received four courses of platinum plus adriamycin and then received maintenance therapy with adriamycin 48 mg/M^2 once a month. However, after remaining in partial

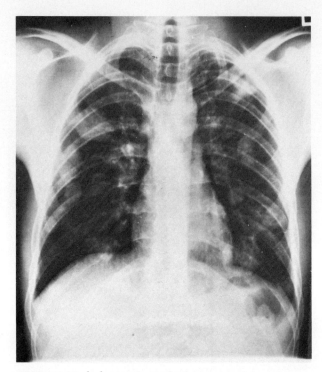

FIGURE 6. Marked regression with platinum + adriamycin chemotherapy.

remission for 4 months, he was readmitted with severe headaches and weakness of his left upper extremity. He was found to have multiple central nervous system metastases and progressive pulmonary metastases. He died 2 weeks later with extensive brain metastases.

Patient 4 was a 25-year-old male with embryonal carcinoma treated initially with orchiectomy and retroperitoneal node dissection. Following surgery, he was placed on chemoprophylaxis with actinomycin-D. However, shortly thereafter, he developed pulmonary metastases, and his chemotherapy was changed to mithramycin. Further progression ensued, and he was then treated with bleomycin, cyclophosphamide, vincristine, methotrexate, and 5-FU (Bleo-COMF). He again failed to respond to this combination regimen, and he was next treated with vinblastine + bleomycin, again with further progression. He was subsequently referred to Indiana University for combination chemotherapy with platinum + adriamycin.

At the time of admission, he had a Karnofsky performance status of 60, and was symptomatic with chest pain, shortness of breath, and dyspnea on exertion. A chest x-ray revealed multiple bilateral pulmonary metastases (Fig. 7). Lactic dehydrogenase (LDH) was markedly elevated (600), but his beta subunit human chorionic gonadotrophin and alpha-fetoprotein levels were both normal.

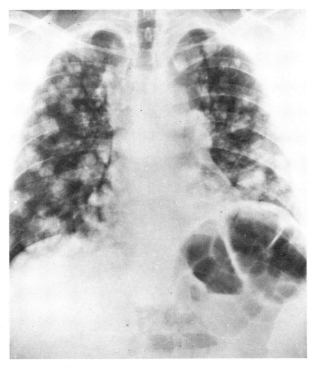

FIGURE 7. Massive pulmonary metastases in patient 4.

He was started on combination chemotherapy with cis-diamminedichloro-platinum 20 mg/M^2 for 5 consecutive days plus adriamycin 60 mg/M^2. He was readmitted 3 weeks later with marked subjective and objective improvement and his LDH decreased to 123. Further improvement was seen with subsequent courses (Fig. 8), and because of continued radiographic regression, he was continued on platinum + adriamycin, receiving a total of seven courses. However, he developed progressive pulmonary metastases after a 5-month partial remission, and died shortly thereafter.

This combination regimen produced nine partial remissions and one complete remission in 10 patients with advanced refractory testicular cancer. Although it was disappointing that we observed only one complete remission, especially when compared to our previous results with cis-diamminedichloroplatinum, vinblastine, and bleomycin, this patient population was a very refractory poor-risk group. In addition to progression on vinblastine plus bleomycin, six patients also had prior radiotherapy, and five patients had also failed on at least one other chemotherapeutic regimen in addition to vinblastine plus bleomycin. In addition, all 10 patients had advanced pulmonary disease and three patients also had advanced abdominal disease. Six patients had teratocarcinoma, and one patient

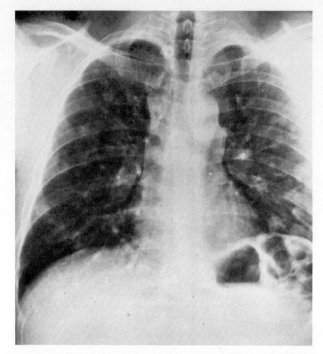

FIGURE 8. Significant regression after one course of platinum adriamycin.

had choriocarcinoma. One of the three embryonal carcinomas was a mediastinal germinoma. Six patients had elevated alpha-fetoprotein levels. All of these factors have been shown to be unfavorable prognostic indicators in previous studies.[18,23,27]

Two other studies have been reported utilizing adriamycin and cis-diam-minedichloroplatinum in a variety of neoplastic diseases. Higby, *et al.* used adriamycin 75 mg/M² plus cis-platinum 20 mg/M² for 5 consecutive days every 28 days, and achieved two complete and one partial remission in three patients with testicular cancer, lasting 5, 10, and 4 months, respectively.[37] These three patients had received prior chemotherapy with actinomycin-D and vinblastine plus bleomycin. Vogl, *et al.* treated five testicular cancer patients with adriamycin 50 mg/M² and platinum 50 mg/M² every 2–3 weeks, and achieved only one partial response in five patients.[38] These numbers are obviously very small, but these two studies, as well as this study, suggest that there may be a therapeutic advantage to 5-day courses of platinum in testicular cancer.

This two-drug regimen produced clinically significant remissions with acceptable toxicity in a very poor-risk patient population. These results were felt to be amply encouraging to warrant investigation of adriamycin as first line

TABLE XII.

R	Platinum 20 mg/M² X 5 days q 3 weeks (3–4 courses)	
A	Bleomycin 30 units IV weekly X 12	
N	Vinblastine *0.4 mg/kg* q 3 weeks	
D	Platinum 20 mg/M² X 5 days q 3 weeks (3–4 courses)	
O	Bleomycin 30 units IV weekly X 12	
M	Vinblastine *0.3 mg/kg* q 3 weeks	
I	Platinum 20 mg/M² X 5 q 3 weeks (3–4 courses)	
Z	Bleomycin 30 units IV weekly X 12	
E	Vinblastine *0.2 mg/kg* q 3 weeks	
	Adriamycin 50 mg/M² q 3 weeks	

After completion of 12 weeks of Bleomycin, maintenance therapy on all three arms to be Vinblastine 0.3 mg/kg monthly for 2 years

chemotherapy in disseminated testicular cancer, in combination with platinum, vinblastine, and bleomycin.

Platinum + Vinblastine + Bleomycin ± Adriamycin

Although platinum + vinblastine + bleomycin as employed at Indiana University has produced very respectable therapeutic results, we have been concerned with the toxicity. Although platinum is potentially nephrotoxic, this has not been a clinical problem since we routinely employ saline hydration. Clinically significant bleomycin pulmonary fibrosis, likewise, is an uncommon complication. Thus, the major serious toxicity has been secondary to high-dose (0.4 mg/kg) vinblastine. Myalgias, constipation, and paralytic ileus were all troublesome side effects, but severe granulocytopenia and potential sepsis was the most worrisome toxicity. Thus, in September 1976, we started a random prospective trial comparing our standard platinum + vinblastine (0.4 mg/kg) + bleomycin with the same regimen using a lowered dosage (0.3 mg/kg) of vinblastine. Also, because of the previously described encouraging results achieved with platinum + adriamycin in patients who failed to respond to vinblastine + bleomycin, a third arm was added to evaluate adriamycin as first line therapy in combination with platinum + vinblastine + bleomycin (Table XII).

Seventy-eight patients have been entered on this study from September 1976 to June 1978, and the results are shown in Table XIII. The complete remission rate (68%) and surgical resection rate for localized residual disease (14%) were remarkably similar to our original platinum + vinblastine + bleomycin study. The relapse rate remains low, and there have been no drug-related deaths. However, one patient died of a pulmonary embolus 3 months after laparotomy for removal of residual embryonal carcinoma. Sixty-five patients (83%) remain alive, and 54 (70%) are alive and continuously disease-free. These patients have

TABLE XIII.
PVB ± Adriamycin Results

	PVB (0.3 mg/kg)	PVB (0.4 mg/kg)	B + adria	Total
No. Patients	27	26	25	78
Complete Remission	17 (63%)	18 (69%)	18 (72%)	53 (68%)
NED with surg.	4 (15%)	5 (19%)	2 (8%)	11 (14%)
Partial Remissions	6 (22%)	3 (12%)	3 (12%)	12 (15%)
Relapses[a]	2 (10%)	4 (17%)	2 (10%)	8 (12%)
Number alive	22 (81%)	23 (88%)	20 (80%)	65 (83%)
Number continuously NED	18 (67%)	19 (73%)	17 (68%)	54 (70%)

[a] Applies only to those patients in CR or NED with surgery.

been followed for a median of 16 months (range 6–27 months).

The effect of prior therapy is shown in Table XIV. In comparison with our original study in which only two of seven patients with prior radiotherapy achieved a complete remission, this patient population had a 73% complete remission rate (11 of 15 patients). The discrepancy is clearly related to a change in our treatment philosophy in patients with prior radiotherapy. As mentioned previously, the vinblastine (and adriamycin) dosages are routinely reduced 25% in such patients. However, even with this dosage reduction, there is still profound and prolonged granulocytopenia in these patients. We now proceed with the second and subsequent courses of platinum combination chemotherapy *on schedule,* rather than waiting for some return of the granulocyte count which often would otherwise delay therapy for several weeks. The second course of platinum + vinblastine + bleomycin is frequently started at a time when the granulocyte count is less then 1000/cc mm. Although this greatly increases the possibility of subsequent granulocytopenic fever and potential sepsis, we feel this is preferable to delaying therapy and losing the initial therapeutic advantage. Despite our present equivalent CR rate in patients with prior radiotherapy, we still feel that radiotherapy should not be employed in patients with nonseminomatous testicular cancer. Although we can now achieve a comparable complete

TABLE XIV.
Prior Therapy and PVB ± Adria

	Numbers	CR	NED + surg.	Presently NED
Surgery alone	52	33 (63%)	9 (17%)	40 (77%)
Prior chemotherapy	17	12 (71%)	1 (6%)	11 (65%)
Prior radiotherapy	15	11 (73%)	1 (7%)	10 (67%)

TABLE XV.
PVB ± Adria and Histology

	Number	CR	NED + surg.	Presently NED
Seminoma	8	6 (75%)	0	6 (75%)
Embryonal	41	31 (76%)	6 (15%)	34 (83%)
Teratocarcinoma	23	16 (70%)	2 (9%)	15 (66%)
Choriocarcinoma	6	0	3 (50%)	3 (50%)

remission rate in such patients, the potential short term toxicity is formidable and perhaps best analogous to remission induction therapy for acute myeloblastic leukemia.

The relationship of histology to response rate is shown in Table XV. There continues to be an extremely high NED rate for embryonal carcinoma, as 37 of 41 patients with this histology achieved a disease-free state (31 with chemotherapy alone and an additional six with surgical removal of residual disease). Although we did not achieve any complete remissions in the six choriocarcinoma patients, three of these patients are presently disease-free after surgical removal of residual abdominal disease after chemotherapeutic clearing of advanced pulmonary disease. Interestingly, we now have a 70% complete remission rate (16 of 23) in teratocarcinoma, compared to 44% (4 of 11 patients) in our original series. However, in that original series, the three patients with prolonged partial remissions (2+ years) all had teratocarcinoma. It is our impression that these chemotherapeutic regimens work equally well in all histologies, with lower CR's in choriocarcinoma because of the larger volume of tumor present at the initiation of chemotherapy.

The most important determinant to achieving complete remission and potential cure remains extent of metastatic disease (Table XVI). Thirty of 31 patients with minimal metastatic disease (categories A, C, and E) achieved complete remission. This emphasizes the importance of the early detection of metastatic disease in

TABLE XVI.
Extent of Disease and PVB ± Adria

	Number	CR	NED + surg.	Presently NED
A. Minimal Pulm	14	13 (93%)	0	11 (79%)
B. Advanced Pulm	20	10 (50%)	3 (15%)	10 (50%)
C. Min. Abd. and Pulm	13	13 (100%)	0	11 (85%)
D. Advanced Abd.	23	10 (43%)	8 (35%)	17 (74%)
E. Elevated markers only	4	4 (100%)	0	4 (100%)
F. Miscellaneous[a]	4	3 (75%)	0	3 (75%)

[a] Two patients with cervical nodes only, one with spinal cord compression and one with bone metastases.

TABLE XVII.
PVB ± Adria and Sepsis

	Granulocytopenic fevers	Documented sepis
PVB (0.3 mg/kg vinblastine)	4 (15%)	0
PVB (0.4 mg/kg vinblastine)	9 (35%)	3 (12%)
PVB + adriamycin	6 (24%)	1 (4%)

patients with Stage I or II disease initially treated with retroperitoneal lymphadenectomy.

The incidence of granulocytopenic fever requiring hospitalization and of documented sepsis is shown in Table XVII. The frequency in the high-dose (0.4 mg/kg) vinblastine arm is almost identical to our original study (38% granulocytopenic fevers and 15% sepsis). The incidence of granulocytopenic fevers and sepsis was significantly reduced in the two arms not employing high-dose vinblastine. The slightly higher incidence of fever in the platinum + vinblastine + bleomycin + adriamycin arm compared to the platinum + low dose vinblastine + bleomycin was possibly related to the higher number of patients with prior radiotherapy in this group.

Multivariate analysis of these 78 patients is shown in Table XVIII. If potential

TABLE XVIII.
Patient Characteristics PVB ± Adria

	PVB (0.4 mg/kg)	PVB (0.3 mg/kg)	PVB + adria
Number of Patients	26	27	25
Extragonadal	1	3	0
Seminoma	3	3	2
Embryonal	14	11	16
Teratocarcinoma	6	11	6
Choriocarcinoma	3	2	1
Prior radiotherapy	4	3	8
Prior chemotherapy	3	4	10
Minimal pulm. mets.	6	5	3
Advanced pulm. mets.	9	3	8
Min. abd. & pulm. mets.	3	3	7
Advanced abd. disease	5	13	5
Elevated markers	2	0	2
Miscellaneous	1[a]	3[a,b,c]	0

[a] Cervical lymphadenopathy only.
[b] Spinal cord compression only.
[c] Bone metastases only.

unfavorable characteristics are analyzed (extent of disease, histology, extragonadal disease, prior therapy), it can be seen that the high-dose vinblastine arm was clearly not overweighed with unfavorable patients. On the basis of this analysis revealing equivalent response rates and survival with reduced toxicity with low-dose vs. high-dose vinblastine when combined with platinum + bleomycin, we no longer recommend our original high-dose vinblastine dosage. The platinum + vinblastine + bleomycin + adriamycin arm had the highest number of patients with both prior radiotherapy and prior chemotherapy. Thus, in June 1978, this three-armed random prospective study was terminated with the recommendation not to pursue high-dose vinblastine in subsequent studies. The other two arms (platinum + 0.3 mg/kg vinblastine + bleomycin vs. platinum + vinblastine + bleomycin + adriamycin) are presently being evaluated both at Indiana University and in the Southeastern Cancer Study Group in a random prospective study.

The role of maintenance therapy in disseminated testicular cancer has never been clearly established. It is quite possible that in a disease where remission induction therapy is so effective and complete remissions can be defined so accurately, maintenance therapy may be unnecessary. A further aspect of the present random prospective study will address this important question, as patients achieving complete remission on either of the two remission induction arms will be randomized to receive maintenance vinblastine (0.3 mg/kg once a month for 20 months) or no further therapy after completion of the 12-week remission induction with platinum combination chemotherapy. All patients in this study will receive four courses of platinum therapy. A historical perspective on this issue was the mithramycin study by Kennedy.[11] In this study, the five patients who achieved complete remission did not receive any form of maintenance therapy after they received 6 months of mithramycin, and none of these patients relapsed.

Adjuvant Therapy

The criteria for successful application of adjuvant therapy is: (1) poor prognosis for cure with primary therapy alone and (2) evidence that the proposed adjuvant therapy is effective in metastatic disease. Stage I nonseminomatous testicular cancer has an 80–100% cure rate with surgery alone, and very few institutions recommend any form of adjuvant therapy. Although such patients are treated and "surgically staged" with a retroperitoneal node dissection, in reality, the only therapy that was necessary was an orchiectomy. Clearly, survival is not enhanced by removal of multiple histologically normal abdominal nodes. Approximately one-half of patients undergoing a retroperitoneal node dissection will be found at surgery to have negative nodes (Stage I). Urologists are cognizant about obtaining whole lung tomograms in their preoperative evaluation to avoid doing unnecessary surgery in patients who already have pulmonary metastases (Stage III disease). However, we also need to direct our attention towards preventing equally unecessary node dissections, with its attendant morbidity including sterility, in patients with Stage I disease. In the past, urologists were legitimately concerned that patients with clinical Stage I disease (normal lymphangiography) might in reality still harbor positive abdominal nodes, and leaving behind such carcinomatous deposits is no longer tenable. First of all, we can more accurately define the patient population that would have a negative node dissection with the availability of radioimmunoassay alpha-fetoprotein and beta subunit human chorionic gonadropin, i.e., those patients with negative markers. Also, abdominal CAT scan and ultrasound enhance our visualization of the retroperitoneum. Patients who have normal HCG, AFP, abdominal ultrasound, and abdominal CAT scan are unlikely to have a positive node dissection. It is probable that about 80–90% of retroperitoneal node dissections on such patients would find only histologically benign nodes. Perhaps in the very near future, as more information is accumulated, the patient population with clinical Stage I disease will *not* receive a radical bilateral retroperitoneal node dissection, but instead will have a staging laparotomy as is done in Hodgkin's disease, with removal of sentinel nodes and other representative nodes, and if such nodes are indeed normal, no further surgery would be required. The other reason why this approach will be feasible is that even if such patients, however rare, do have "missed" carcinomatous retroperitoneal nodes, that does not condemn the patient to subsequent progression and ultimate death. These patients would still have close follow-up, with monthly HCG, AFP, and chest x-rays once a month for 1 year, and every other month the second year of observation. Should recurrent disease become manifest, the probability of cure with effective chemotherapy should be exceedingly high. At Indiana University, we are currently doing bilateral retroperitoneal node dissections on all patients with clinical Stage I or II disease, and all such patients have preoperative abdominal ultrasound, abdominal CAT scan, and HCG and AFP determinations. We will then retrospectively analyze the data to determine how many clinical Stage I patients (markers and radiographic studies negative) converted to surgical Stage II disease with retroperitoneal lymphadenectomy.

Patients with Stage II disease have a considerably more ominous prognosis for surgical cure. Generally speaking, patients with microscopically positive nodes, and fewer than five in number, will have a 60–80% cure rate with surgery alone. Patients with grossly positive nodes surgically resected have only a 20–60% cure rate with surgery alone. Obviously, the bulkier the retroperitoneal involvement, and the more positive nodes found pathologically, the worse the prognosis.

Although adjuvant chemotherapy for patients with Stage II disease appears attractive, and clearly would reduce the surgical relapse rate, it may not be capable of improving survival, as it should approach 100% in properly managed patients treated with retroperitoneal lymphadenectomy. Although a high percentage of Stage II patients will ultimately relapse, such patients are imminently curable with present day chemotherapy administered at the time of relapse. Postoperative patients with testicular cancer should be followed monthly the first year and every other month the second year with physical examination, HCG,

AFP, and chest x-ray. This method of follow-up should help to assure that when the patient relapses, he will do so with "minimal" metastatic disease, and patients with minimal metastatic disease and no prior chemotherapy or radiotherapy have an expected 95–100% complete remission rate with platinum combination chemotherapy, with a very low subsequent relapse rate. Postoperative radiotherapy for such patients probably does not decrease the relapse rate, and may be deleterious because of inability to give full dose chemotherapy at the time of relapse. Radiotherapy instead of retroperitoneal lymphadenectomy may be capable of producing equivalent results in selected patients with Stage I or Stage II disease. Sandwich radiotherapy (preoperative irradiation, retroperitoneal lymphadenectomy, and postoperative irradiation) may be capable of minimally improving the results obtained with surgery alone. However, 10–20% of Stage I and 20–60% of Stage II patients will ultimately relapse after initial therapy, and those patients that received prior radiotherapy may be in a distinct disadvantage because of the difficulty in administering subsequent curative chemotherapy.

It is somewhat surprising that actinomycin-D, a drug shown to be effective in Stage III non-seminomatous testicular cancer 20 years ago, has never been tested in a random prospective study as a surgical adjuvant in Stage II disease. Ansfield and Ramirez reported on the use of adjuvant triple therapy with actinomycin-D plus chlorambucil plus methotrexate in an uncontrolled study.[39] This therapy was delivered as an adjuvant to surgery in 32 patients (4 choriocarcinoma, 17 embryonal, and 11 teratocarcinoma). However, about one-third of these patients had Stage I disease. Nevertheless, the results were noteworthy with 24 of 32 patients (75%) alive and disease-free for over 3 years.

The Memorial group, again in an uncontrolled study, treated 60 patients with Stage II nonseminomatous testicular cancer with adjuvant chemotherapy following orchiectomy and retroperitoneal dissection. These patients received "mini-VAB," consisting of actinomycin-D 0.02 mg/kg IV, vinblastine 0.06 mg/kg IV and bleomycin 0.25 mg/kg IV weekly for 6 weeks, then actinomycin-D 0.02 mg/kg IV followed with chlorambucil 0.15 mg/kg p.o. for 7 days every 2–3 weeks for 2–3 years.[40] The initial results (with a short follow-up) looked favorable, with only 11 relapses (18%). However, a more recent up-date with longer follow-up revealed that approximately 50% of those patients with grossly positive nodes have relapsed.[41]

We have followed 112 patients with Stage I or II nonseminomatous testicular cancer treated with orchiectomy followed by a bilateral retroperitoneal lymphadenectomy. These patients have been followed from 4 to 65 months with a median of 28 months. There were 57 surgical Stage I patients in this series and none of these patients received postoperative therapy. Four (7%) have relapsed; however, they all went into complete remission with platinum + vinblastine + bleomycin, and all 57 Stage I patients are presently alive and disease-free. There were 55 Stage II patients, and 26 of those patients had grossly positive nodes. Eighteen patients (33%) have relapsed. Initially, it was our treatment policy to treat surgical Stage II patients with monthly courses of actinomycin-D for 1 year following lymphadenectomy. Thirty-one patients were given adjuvant actinomycin-D, and 14 relapsed (45%). However, these 14 patients then received platinum + vinblastine + bleomycin for recurrent Stage III disease, and all achieved complete remission. One of these Stage III patients later relapsed and subsequently succumbed to metastatic testicular cancer. As our experience with platinum + vinblastine + bleomycin for Stage III disease increased, and the therapeutic results became apparent, we discontinued adjuvant actinomycin-D. Our primary treatment philosophy in the past several years for Stage II disease has been to administer *NO* adjuvant chemotherapy, but instead follow such patients at monthly intervals for the first postoperative year with HCG, AFP, and chest x-ray, and obtain the same studies every 2 months the second year of observation. Twenty-four patients with Stage II disease were thus followed and four have relapsed. However, all of these patients again achieved complete remission with platinum + vinblastine + bleomycin.

In 1977–1978, seven patients with grossly positive nodes received adjuvant chemotherapy with platinum 20 mg/M^2 × 5 days every 3 weeks for two courses plus vinblastine 0.3 mg/kg every 3 weeks for two dosages plus bleomycin 30 units IV push weekly for 6 weeks, and all seven of these patients remain disease-free. This was done as a pilot study for a proposed intergroup national adjuvant chemotherapy study for Stage II nonseminomatous testicular cancer.

Clearly, the only way to determine the value of adjuvant platinum combination chemotherapy would be with a carefully designed random prospective clinical trial. As mentioned above, our experience at Indiana has primarily been without aggressive adjuvant chemotherapy, and 111 of 112 patients are presently alive and disease-free. This data reemphasizes our belief that the cure rate for properly managed Stage I and Stage II disease should approach 100%. Our primary philosophy to achieve this goal is:

1. Monthly follow-up for 1 year post-retroperitoneal lymphadenectomy (whether Stage I or II) with HCG, AFP, and chest x-ray, and the same studies every 2 months during the second year of observation. Surgical relapses beyond this point are uncommon, and the same studies should be done only every 4–6 months thereafter.
2. Avoid preoperative and/or postoperative radiotherapy in nonseminomatous testicular cancer, as this will compromise chemotherapy and increase drug morbidity and mortality in those patients who relapse and subsequently require chemotherapy.
3. Use effective chemotherapy if and when recurrent disease becomes manifest.

Conclusion

There is no longer any justification for pessimism in the management of patients with disseminated testicular cancer, and such patients *must* be treated with curative intent. Platinum + vinblastine + bleomycin consistently produces 70% complete remissions, and a further 10% of patients will be rendered disease-free following surgical excision of residual disease. The relapse rate in such patients remains low (10–20%), and all relapses have occurred within 9 months of initiation of complete remission, except for one late relapse at 17 months. Toxicity with the lower dosage (0.3 mg/kg) of vinblastine is considerably less than with the higher dosage (0.4 mg/kg), with an equivalent therapeutic response. We no longer recommend high-dose vinblastine as part of the platinum + vinblastine + bleomycin regimen. We are still evaluating the role (if any) of the addition of adriamycin and of maintenance therapy with vinblastine.

The projected cure rate for patients today with Stage III nonseminomatous testicular cancer is 60–70%. It is interesting to note that this is higher than the *surgical* cure rate for Stage II disease. Major progress has clearly been made in the past decade in disseminated testicular cancer, as the projected cure rate in the 1960's was less than 10%. Platinum plus vinblastine plus bleomycin represents a major advance in the treatment of testicular cancer.

References

1. Mackay, E. N., and Sellers A. H.: A statistical review of malignant testicular tumors based on the experience of the Ontario Cancer Foundation Clinics, 1938, 1961. *Can Med Assoc J* **94**:889–899, 1966.

2. Maier, J. G., Mittemyer, B. T., and Sulak, M. H.: Treatment and prognosis in seminoma of the testis. *J Urol* **99**:72–78, 1968.

3. Freedman, M., and Purkayastha, M. C.: Recurrent seminoma: management of late metastases, recurrence of a second primary tumor. *Am J Roentgenol Radium Ther Nucl Med* **83**:25–42, 1960.

4. Lange, P. H., McIntire, K. R., Waldmann, T. A., *et al.*: Serum alpha fetoprotein and human chorionic gonadotropin in the diagnosis and management of non-seminomatous germ-cell testicular cancer. *N Engl J Med* **295**:1237–1240, 1976.

5. Donohue, J. P.: Retroperitoneal lymphadenectomy—The anterior approach including bilateral suprarenal-hilar dissection. *Urol Clin North Am* **4**:509–523, 1977.

6. Javadpour, N., McIntire, R. K., Waldman, T. A., Scardino, P. T., Bergman, S., and Anderson, T.: The role of the radioimmunoassay of serum alphafetoprotein and human chorionic gonadotropin in the intensive chemotherapy and surgery of metastatic testicular tumors. *J Urol* **119**:759–762, 1978.

7. Li, M. C., Whitmore, W. F., Golbey, R., and Grabstad, H.: Effects of combined drug therapy on metastatic cancer of the testis. *J Am Med Assoc* **174**:145–153, 1960.

8. Ansfield, F. J., Korbitz, B. D., Davis, H. L., Jr., Ramirez, G.: Triple therapy in testicular tumors. *Cancer* **24**:442–446, 1969.

9. MacKenzie, A. R.: Chemotherapy of metastatic testis cancer—results in 154 patients. *Cancer* **19**:1369–1376, 1966.

10. Samuels, M. L., and Howe, C. D.: Vinblastine in the management of testicular cancer. *Cancer* **25**:1009–1017, 1970.

11. Kennedy, B. J.: Mithramycin therapy in advanced testicular neoplasms. *Cancer* **26**:755–766, 1970.

12. Blum, R. H., Carter, S., and Agre, K.: A clinical review of bleomycin—a new antineoplastic agent. *Cancer* **31**:903–914, 1973.

13. Wyatt, J. K., and McAninch, L. H.: A chemotherapeutic approach to advanced testicular carcinoma. *Can J Surg* **10**:421–426, 1967.

14. Mendelson, D., and Serpick, A. A.: Combination chemotherapy of testicular tumors. *J Urol* **103**:619–623, 1970.

15. DeVita, V., Canellos, G., Hubbard, S., Chabner, B., and Young, R.: Chemotherapy of Hodgkin's disease with MOPP: A 10 year progress report. *Proc Am Soc Clin Oncol* **17**:269, 1976 (abstract).

16. Samuels, M. L., Johnson, D. E., and Holoye, P. Y.: Continuous intravenous bleomycin (NSC-125066) therapy with vinblastine (NSC-49842) in stage III testicular neoplasia. *Cancer Chemother Rep* **59**:563–570, 1975.

17. Samuels, M. L., Lanzotti, V. J., Holoye, P. Y., Boyle, L. E., Smith, T. L., and Johnson, D. E.: Combination chemotherapy in germinal cell tumors. *Cancer Treat Rev* **3**:185–204, 1976.

18. Samuels, M. L., Lanzotti, V. J., Holoye, P. Y., and Howe, C. D.: Stage III testicular cancer: complete response by substage to velban plus continuous bleomycin infusion (VB-3). *Proc Am Assoc Cancer Res* **18**:146, 1977.

19. Barranco, S. C., and Humphrey, R. M.: The effects of bleomycin on survival and cell progression in Chinese hamster cells in vitro. *Cancer Res* **31**:1218–1223, 1971.

20. Rosenberg, B., VanCamp, L., and Krigas, T.: Inhibition of cell division in E. coli by electrolysis products from a platinum electrode. *Nature* **205**:678–699, 1965.

21. Higby, D. J., Wallace, H. J., Albert, D. J., and Holland, J. F.: Diaminodichloroplatinum: a phase I study showing responses in testicular and other tumors. *Cancer* **33**:1219–1225, 1974.

22. Wittes, R. E., Yagoda, A., Silvay, O., Magill, G. B., Whitmore, W. Krakoff, I. H., and Golbey, R. B.: Chemotherapy of germ cell tumors of the testis. *Cancer* **37**:637–645, 1976.

23. Cvitkovic, E., Cheng, E., Whitmore, W. F., and Golbey, R. B.: Germ cell tumor chemotherapy update. *Proc. Am Soc Clin Oncol* **18**:324, 1977.

24. Cvitkovic, E., Wittes, R., Golbey, R., and Krakoff, I. H.: Primary combination chemotherapy (VAB II) for metastatic or unresectable germ cell tumors. *Proc Am Assoc Cancer Res* **19**:174, 1978.

25. Cheng, E., Cvitkovic, E., Wittes, R. E., and Golby, R. B.: Germ cell tumors: VAB II in metastatic testicular cancer. *Cancer* **42**:2162–2168, 1978.

26. Intergroup Cooperative Study of Testicular Cancer, Chicago, May, 1978.

27. Einhorn, L. H., and Donohue, J. P.: Cis-diamminedichloroplatinum, vinblastine, and bleomycin combination chemotherapy in disseminated testicular cancer. *Ann Intern Med* **87**:293–298, 1977.

28. Willis, G. W., and Hajdu, S. I.: Histologically benign teratoid metastasis of testicular embryonal carcinoma: report of five cases. *Am J Clin Pathol* **59**:388–343, 1973.

29. Merrin, C., Takita, H., Weber, R., Wagsman, Z., Baugartner, G., and Murphy, G. P.: Combination radical surgery and multiple sequential chemotherapy for the treatment of advanced carcinoma of the testis (stage III). *Cancer* **37**:20–29, 1976.

30. Hong, W. K., Wittes, R. E., Hajdu, S. T., Cvitkovic, E., Witmore, W. F., and Golbey, R. B.: The evolution of mature teratoma from malignant testicular tumors. *Cancer* **40**: 2987–2992, 1977.

31. Johnson, D. E., Bracken, R. B., Ayala, A. G., and Samuels, M. L.: Retroperitoneal lymphadenecotmy as adjunctive therapy in selected cases of advanced testicular carcinoma. *J Urol* **116**:66–68, 1976.

32. Dentino, M., Luft, F. C., Yum, M. N., Williams, S. D., and Einhorn, L. H.: Long term effect of cis-diamminedichloride platinum (CDDP) on renal function and structure in man. *Cancer* **41**:1274–1281, 1978.

33. Stark, J. J., and Howell S. B.: Nephrotoxicity of cis-platinum dichlorodiammine. *Clin. Pharmacol Ther* **23**:461–465, 1978.

34. Samson, M. K., and Stephens, R. L.: Vinblastine, bleomycin, and cis-diamminedichloroplatinum in disseminated testicular cancer. *Proc. Am Assoc Cancer Res* **19**:12, 1978.

35. Einhorn, L. H., and Williams, S. D.: Combination chemotherapy with cis-diamminedi-chloroplatinum and adriamycin in testicular cancer refractory to vinblastine plus bleomycin. *Cancer Treat Rep* **62**:1351–1353, 1978.

36. Monfardini, S., Bajetta, E., Musumeci, R., *et al.*: Clinical use of adriamycin in advanced testicular cancer. *J Urol* **108**:293–296, 1972.

37. Higby, D. J., Wilbur, D., Wallace, H. J., *et al.*: Adriamycin-cyclophosphamide and ad-riamycin-cis-dichlorodiammineplatinum combination chemotherapy in patients with advanced cancer. *Cancer Treat Rep* **61**:869–873, 1977.

38. Vogl, S., Ohnuma, T., Perloff, M., *et al.*: Combination chemotherapy with adriamycin and cis-diamminedichloroplatinum in patients with neoplastic disease. *Cancer* **38**:21–26, 1976.

39. Ansfield, F. J., and Ramirez, G.: Triple therapy as an adjuvant to testicular cancer surgery. International Conference on the Adjuvant Therapy of Cancer, Tucson, Arizona, 1977 (abstract).

40. Vugrin, D., Cvitkovic, E., Whitmore, W., and Golbey, R. B.: Prophylactic chemotherapy of testicular germ cell carcinomas (nonseminomas) Stage II following orchiectomy and retroperitoneal dissection. *Proc. Am Soc Clin Oncol* **19**:352, 1978.

41. Cvitkovic, E.: Statement made at Genitourinary Oncology Symposium, Houston, Texas, November 1978.

7

Chemotherapy of
Metastatic Seminoma *

Lawrence H. Einhorn, M.D.

*Department of Medicine, Indiana University Medical Center and Veterans'
Administration Hospital, Indianapolis, Indiana*

IN THE 1960S AND 1970S, major controversy erupted concerning the optimal
management of nonseminomatous testicular cancer. During this same time period, it was frequently stated that one reason for this controversy was the unsat-
isfactory survival data for nonseminomatous tumors compared to seminoma. Stage
I seminoma has a 95–100% cure rate with radiotherapy and Stage II an 80–95%
cure rate, and the results were far superior to that achieved in nonseminomatous
tumors.

However, an abrupt about-face is presently occurring, mainly due to extremely
effective chemotherapy. In the 1980s the proper management of Stage II and
III seminoma will be a major area of controversy because the cure rate for nonseminomatous tumors may well exceed that for pure seminoma. Radiotherapists
define Stage III seminoma as lymphatic supradiaphragmatic involvement
(mediastinal and/or cervical nodes), and Stage IV disease as visceral involvement
(hepatic, osseous, pulmonary, central nervous system). These definitions will be
utilized during the remainder of this chapter.

The purpose of this chapter is to put into perspective present or future areas
of controversy concerning the management of patients with seminoma.

* Supported in part by PHS Grant M01 RROO 750-06.

151

Stage I and II Typical Seminoma

The percentage of testicular tumors represented by seminoma varies with the population under study, ranging from 35 to 70%. Generally speaking, these patients are 10–20 years older than patients with nonseminomatous tumors, with the peak age group in the fourth and fifth decades.[1]

Pure seminoma is an exquisitely radiosensitive neoplasm that has an orderly lymphatic spread. High cure rates are regularly achieved with orchiectomy and appropriate irradiation, and retroperitoneal node dissection is rarely indicated.[2] The true incidence of occult retroperitoneal nodes in patients with clinical Stage I seminoma (negative lymphangiogram and/or abdominal ultrasound and computed tomography) is usually unknown because these patients are not subjected to surgical staging. Nevertheless, patients with clinical Stage I seminoma are routinely treated with orchiectomy plus elective regional lymphatic irradiation because about 10–20% of lymphangiograms are falsely negative.[3] Standard therapy for clinical Stage I seminoma is a tumor dose of 2500 rad in 3 weeks to the periaortic and ipsilateral iliac areas. Hussey and Doornbos utilized this therapeutic strategy and only one patient developed metastatic disease in the mediastinal or supraclavicular areas. Their 3-year disease-free survival was 95.2% (59 of 62 patients).[5]

These authors do not feel "prophylactic" irradiation to the mediastinum and left supraclavicular fossa is necessary in clinical Stage I seminoma. Interestingly, 20 patients were treated by these authors with the addition of mediastinal and supraclavicular irradiation, and, although none developed recurrent seminoma, two patients subsequently died from acute leukemia.[5] Other authors also report a 95–100% cure rate with orchiectomy plus irradiation for Stage I seminoma.[6–8]

Fortunately, approximately 65% of patients with seminoma present as Stage I disease.[5–8] Because of the outstanding results achieved, there is very little rationale for controversy in the therapeutic management of Stage I seminoma. The cure rate for clinical Stage II (positive lymphangiogram or palpable abdominal mass) is still excellent, but does not approach the 95–100% salvage rate attained in Stage I disease. Most authors report a 75–90% cure rate.[5–8] Several authors have subdivided Stage II disease into two separate categories; IIA implies involved retroperitoneal nodes per intravenous pyelogram and/or lymphangiogram, and IIB denotes palpable abdominal disease. As expected, the radiocurability of Stage IIB is worse than that observed for Stage IIA, but, nevertheless, Hussey reported 7 of 12 (58.3%) such patients disease-free after a minimum of 36 months follow-up,[5] and Cionini salvaged 16 of 23 (70%) Stage IIB patients with orchiectomy plus radiotherapy. Prophylactic irradiation to the mediastinum and left supraclavicular fossa is routinely added to the abdominal radiotherapy for patients with Stage IIA and IIB. Although some authors suggest the use of adjuvant chemotherapy with an alkylating agent (usually chlorambucil), it is my opinion that patients with Stage IIA or IIB seminoma should still be treated with radiotherapy alone. However, such patients should be followed every 4–8 weeks for at least 2 years after initiation of radiotherapy, as 90% of recurrences occur within 2 years.[8] When a relapse occurs, it should be treated with further radiotherapy[9] or chemotherapy, depending upon the nature of the relapse.

Stage III Seminoma

Stage III seminoma is defined as lymphatic involvement above the diaphragm (cervical and/or mediastinal nodes). This is separate from Stage IV disease, as defined by most radiotherapists. Stage IV disease is visceral involvement and usually implies pulmonary, osseous, and/or hepatic involvement.

There is not a large amount of information available in the literature concerning the proper management of Stage III seminoma. Furthermore, this accounts for only 5% of all clinical presentations of seminoma. The cure rate with radiotherapy for Stage III disease has been dismal.[6–8] Only Hussey[5] has reported a salvage rate above 40% (three of five alive and disease-free at 3 years). Furthermore, since the majority of these patients will relapse following an abortive attempt for radiocurability, they will then require chemotherapy. Prior mediastinal irradiation compromises the safe administration of bleomycin due to an increased probability of pulmonary fibrosis. Virtually all chemotherapy series report major difficulty delivering effective dosages of myelosuppressive agents in such patients without life-threatening hematological toxicity. Although there is no large series utilizing chemotherapy as initial therapy for Stage III seminoma, it is my belief that such patients should receive platinum + vinblastine + bleomycin as first-line therapy, and radiotherapy should be reserved to consolidate the remission if necessary; i.e., if only a partial remission is achieved (clinically or radiographically), appropriate radiotherapy should then be administered. Note is made of the fact that such previously untreated patients with Stage III seminoma will usually present as minimal metastatic disease by chemotherapy standards, unless a large palpable retroperitoneal mass is an accompaniment. Our chemotherapy experience with platinum + vinblastine + bleomycin in testicular cancer patients with minimal metastatic disease indicates a 90–100% probability for achieving a complete remission and only a 15% probability of relapse (see chapter on management of disseminated testicular cancer). Since our response rate with this chemotherapy program for seminoma is similar to that seen in nonseminomatous disease (*vide infra*), it is not unreasonable to expect at least an 80% cure rate with chemotherapy alone in Stage III seminoma. Furthermore, those patients not salvaged by chemotherapy alone may still be curable with postchemotherapy irradiation.

Anaplastic Seminoma

This histologic variant accounts for 10% of all seminomas. Most authors feel that anaplastic seminoma is a more virulent disease than typical seminoma, but

Maier feels that the poorer therapeutic results are primarily due to the advanced stage at presentation.[4] In Maier's series, 17 of 18 patients with Stage I or II anaplastic seminoma were cured with radiotherapy. However, Kademian and coauthors salvaged only two of four Stage I anaplastic seminomas, and overall, only five of eight anaplastic seminomas remain alive at two, four, 36, 48, and 120 months.[10] Similarly, Johnson, Gomez, and Ayala noted only three of seven survivors with anaplastic seminoma.[11]

Despite the apparent decreased survival with anaplastic seminoma, I still feel that radiotherapy alone is adequate therapy for clinical Stage I or II disease. However, there is no role for radiotherapy as initial therapy in Stage III anaplastic seminoma. Kademian points out that "no report of a cure of a Stage III anaplastic seminoma could be found in the literature."[10] Such patients should have an excellent cure rate with platinum + vinblastine + bleomycin (*vide infra*), especially as first-line therapy rather than being employed after extensive radiotherapy.

Elevated HCG and Alphafetoprotein in Seminoma

The availability of serum radioimmunoassay human chorionic gonadotropin (HCG) and alpha-fetoprotein (AFP) have greatly improved the diagnostic and therapeutic management of germinal neoplasms. These two valuable serum markers are discussed in excellent detail by Dr. Lange, *et al.* in a separate chapter. The value and significance of elevated HCG and/or AFP in nonseminomatous testicular cancer is indisputable. However, the significance of these elevated markers in patients with pure seminoma has been a matter of some controversy.

On the basis of clinical experience[12] and the present understanding of the cellular origin of AFP,[13,14] it appears that an elevated level in a patient with seminoma clearly indicates the presence of nonseminomatous elements. To my knowledge, there has never been a well-documented case of pure seminoma in which the AFP was elevated but no nonseminomatous tumor could be found, either initially by serial sectioning of the orchiectomy specimen, or subsequently with the development of nonseminomatous metastases. Therefore, all patients with a diagnosis of seminoma must have a serum alpha-fetoprotein by radioimmunoassay, and those rare patients with an elevated AFP should be managed in the same manner as a nonseminomatous tumor for that particular stage. Other authors have made similar observations and conclusions.[15,16]

Similar dogmatic conclusions cannot be made concerning the significance of an elevated HCG in a patient with pure seminoma. Earlier reports suggested that an elevated HCG in such patients is definitive evidence for the presence of extragonadal nonseminomatous elements (or elements of nonseminoma by serial sectioning or cellular localization techniques of the orchiectomy specimen).[16,17] This opinion was bolstered by autopsy data indicating that about 1/3 of patients dying of seminoma had nonseminomatous metastases,[4,18] and the fact that 38% of patients with metastatic seminoma had elevated HCG levels.[19] However, there have been some patients with seminoma and elevated HCG levels that have clearly been cured by orchiectomy and irradiation alone.[20] This does not prove that these patients had pure seminoma, however, as they may have had Stage I or early Stage II disease with some nonseminomatous elements, which, of course, can be cured by orchiectomy and radiotherapy alone.[21]

The seminoma study group accumulated data on 31 patients with seminoma and elevated AFP and/or HCG.[20] Four patients had elevated AFP, and all had nonseminomatous elements (one in testis and three subsequently in metastatic lesions). Three patients had minimal elevation of HCG with normal AFP, and these patients were all cured with orchiectomy plus irradiation. A further five patients had clinical Stage I seminoma with an elevated HCG only before orchiectomy that returned to normal prior to initiation of irradiation. These five patients all remain disease-free for 2+ years following orchiectomy and radiotherapy. Another five patients presented with clinical Stage II seminoma; these patients all had a return to normal of their elevated HCG levels following radiotherapy; and all five remain disease-free. However, there were eight similar patients with Stage II seminoma initially treated with orchiectomy plus irradiation who subsequently relapsed and died despite the subsequent administration of chemotherapy. All investigators noted great difficulty in administering chemotherapy because of the prior irradiation. Finally, there was a very interesting group of three patients with pure seminoma, elevated HCG and normal AFP, and advanced metastatic disease treated *initially* with chemotherapy (platinum + vinblastine + bleomycin). Those three patients all achieved complete remission with chemotherapy alone, and all remain alive and disease-free for 2+ years.

What conclusions can be made concerning patients with pure seminoma and elevated markers, and how certain can one be that these conclusions are accurate?

1. Patients with pure seminoma and elevated AFP should be treated in a similar manner as their nonseminomatous counterparts—definite conclusion.
2. Patients with pure Stage I or II seminoma, normal AFP, and minimal elevation (less than 20 mIU/ml) of HCG should be treated with appropriate radiotherapy—definite conclusion.
3. Patients with anaplastic seminoma Stage I or II and elevated HCG should be treated with retroperitoneal lymphadenectomy—personal opinion of the author.
4. Patients with Stage III anaplastic seminoma (with or without elevated HCG) should be treated with platinum combination chemotherapy—definite conclusion.
5. Patients with Stage III seminoma (lymphatic involvement above the diaphragm) and an elevated HCG should be treated with platinum combination chemotherapy—definite conclusion.
6. Patients with clinical Stage I or II seminoma with HCG levels above 20 mIU/ml constitute the most difficult patient population as there are no firm guidelines for management. It is my personal belief that such patients should usually be managed with retroperitoneal lymphadenectomy rather than irradiation, although that point is clearly debatable, especially in those patients with HCG levels below 100 mIU/ml. The issue is not whether radiotherapy can cure this variety of disease, but whether

it is the best method of treatment. Because of data indicating a relatively high relapse rate in such patients treated with irradiation, and the subsequent difficulty in administration of chemotherapy after recurrence, I favor the surgical approach for such patients as initial therapy.

Chemotherapy of Metastatic Seminoma

A discussion on the chemotherapy of metastatic seminoma must begin with the realization that what appears to be metastatic seminoma may in reality be nonseminomatous disease. Patients who were initially treated with orchiectomy and irradiation for pure seminoma and later develop metastases may possibly have a different cell type than their original presentation, and most metastases are not rebiopsied, especially osseous or pulmonary metastases. This concept is further supported by the evidence that approximately 1/3 of all patients dying of "metastatic seminoma" in reality also have nonseminomatous elements.[4,18] The significance of elevated AFP and HCG has already been discussed, but it is worth reiterating that, in Braunstein's series, 38% of patients with metastatic seminoma had elevated HCG levels.[19] It is thus very difficult to determine whether metastatic seminoma is or is not a unique type of germ cell tumor and should have a separate plan of chemotherapy strategy compared to metastatic nonseminomatous germ-cell tumors.

Most of the earlier single-agent chemotherapy trials in metastatic seminoma were done at a time when radioimmunoassay AFP and HCG were not available, and, thus, little or no marker data were available for these patients. Alkylating agents were considered to be "radiomimetic" and therefore were a logical foundation for the chemotherapy of metastatic seminoma. Even with the reservations listed above, there is little reason to believe that alkylating agents have specificity in seminoma compared to their activity in other cell types and even less evidence to suggest that they should be the chemotherapeutic agent of choice today in metastatic seminoma. During the past 20 years, most chemotherapy programs that were successful in nonseminomatous tumors had a similar response rate in metastatic seminoma, taking into account the fact that the latter patients were in a worse prognostic category because of their prior radiotherapy. This is especially true in those few patients treated initially with chemotherapy rather than radiotherapy for metastatic seminoma.[20]

Alkylating Agents in Seminoma

Alkylating agents have become the accepted standard for the treatment of seminomas relapsing after radiotherapy. The reason for the early preference for alkylating agents was the concept that these drugs were "radiomimetic" and the high level of radiocurability of seminoma. However, some of these early studies included patients relapsing in irradiated fields, and obviously the concept of a radiomimetic agent being preferential in such a clinical situation is illogical. In all probability, some of these radiorecurrent tumors represented nonseminomatous tumors.

The largest series ever published is the Russian experience with the alkylating agent sarcolysin. Chebotareva obtained a 90% (38/42) response rate with sarcolysin.[22,23] Although these results are laudable, interpretation of the data has been very tenuous. It seems that many, if not most, of these patients were clinical Stage II seminoma treated with sarcolysin instead of irradiation,[23] and the author's comment that "nodal metastases were especially sensitive, but pulmonary metastases were less sensitive."[23] Furthermore, the experience at Memorial with sarcolysis, although anecdotal, failed to reveal any remission in either of the two patients studied.[24]

The American experience with single-agent alkylators is considerably more sparse. Snyder reported two patients with metastatic seminoma treated with cyclophosphamide, with one brief remission, and one complete remission for 13+ months. MacKenzie reported the initial Memorial experience with chlorambucil,[25,26] a drug that has subsequently become one of the most widely used agents in metastatic seminoma. Chlorambucil was given in a dosage of 10 mg/day orally for 13–66 consecutive days; repeat courses were then given every other month. Four patients with metastatic seminoma were treated, and two partial and two complete remissions were obtained. One complete remission (osseous metastases) relapsed and the other complete remission (pulmonary metastases) remained disease-free for 20 months at the time of MacKenzie's publication.[25] This latter patient did not have prior radiotherapy. MacKenzie also studied chlorambucil in four patients with nonseminomatous metastases, but no responses were observed,[25] suggesting the possibility that alkylators may be more effective in seminoma than nonseminomatous tumors. However, these numbers are very small, and one study employing high-dose cyclophosphamide demonstrated two complete and six partial remissions in nine patients with disseminated nonseminomatous testicular cancer.[27] Interestingly, MacKenzie also observed two of three partial remissions of pulmonary metastases with actinomycin-D as a single agent in metastatic testicular cancer and two of four partial remissions with actinomycin-D + chlorambucil + methotrexate combination chemotherapy.[25] These early studies, in which only a single patient achieved a durable remission, laid the foundation for the widespread usage of alkylating agents in metastatic seminoma.[25,26]

Whitmore has recently updated the Memorial experience with chemotherapy in metastatic seminoma.[24] This is the largest published American series, consisting of 18 testicular seminomas and four mediastinal seminomas. It is interesting to note that only three of these patients had no prior radiotherapy, and two achieved complete remission and remain disease-free with chemotherapy. One of these patients presented with clinical Stage III seminoma with a positive lymphangiogram and mediastinal and supraclavicular nodes. This patient achieved a complete remission with chlorambucil as initial therapy (following orchiectomy) and has remained free of disease for over 5 years. The second patient (with no prior radiotherapy) was a patient with a primary mediastinal seminoma with axillary and cervical nodes. This patient was cured with actinomycin-D +

chlorambucil and received a total of 9 years of maintenance chemotherapy. The only other complete remission with chemotherapy alone was in a patient who presented initially with Stage I seminoma treated with orchiectomy and abdominal irradiation. Less than 1 year after completion of radiotherapy, a mediastinal mass developed and the patient then received 5 years of chlorambucil with a continuous complete remission.

Two other patients in Whitmore's series also were rendered free of disease, but with chemotherapy + radiotherapy. One of these was a patient with Stage II seminoma who achieved a complete remission with chlorambucil + actinomycin-D and then received "adjuvant radiotherapy to the abdomen and mediastinum." This patient has remained free of disease for 4+ years. A second patient had far-advanced metastatic seminoma with bilateral pulmonary metastases and osseous metastases. His pulmonary lesions disappeared with a single dose of nitrogen mustard (!) and never recurred, and he also received radiotherapy to the spine and has remained free of disease for over 9 years.

These were the only complete responses in this series. The entire tabulation of drug trials in this patient population is shown in Table I. It should be noted that the 22% complete and 22% partial response rate with chlorambucil is very similar to results reported during a similar time period with actinomycin-D alone in nonseminomatous testicular cancer.[25] Overall, there were three complete (20%) and three partial (20%) responses with alkylating agents in metastatic seminoma. Furthermore, alkylating agents were a part of a combination regimen in 10 trials, and two complete (20%) and two partial (20%) responses were again obtained. This data demonstrates activity of alkylating agents in seminoma but does not create a mandate for their preferential use over other active drugs in testicular cancer.

TABLE I.
Chemotherapy in Seminoma—The Memorial Experience[24]

Drug Regimen	No. patients	CR	PR
chlorambucil (CLB)	9	2 (22%)	2 (22%)
nitrogen mustard	3	1[a] (33%)	1 (33%)
L-sarcolysin	2	0	0
thiotepa	1	0	0
mithramycin	1	0	0
vincristine	2	0	0
vinblastine + cyclophosphamide	1	0	0
CLB + actino-D	4	2[a] (50%)	0
CLB + actino-D + methotrexate	3	0	1 (33%)
COMF[b]	2	0	1 (50%)

[a] One patient received radiotherapy as well as chemotherapy
[b] Cyclophosphamide (or chlorambucil) + vincristine + methotrexate + 5-FU

TABLE II.
Single Agents (Non-Alkylators) in Metastatic Seminoma

Drug	No. patients	CR	PR	Reference
5-fluorouracil	6	0	3	28–31
actinomycin-D	3	0	2	25
vinblastine	8	0	3	32–33
mithramycin	29	0	9	34–38
adriamycin	4	1	2	39
platinum	5	4	0	40–41

The authors also stated that there were fewer favorable responses to chemotherapy following extensive prior radiotherapy, and there was only one complete remission with chemotherapy alone in patients with prior radiotherapy. Although the complete remissions were significant, Whitmore states that "the three complete remissions achieved with chemotherapy alone might have been achieved with radiotherapy alone."[24]

There have been very few reported results of other single agents in metastatic seminoma, and these are listed in Table II. The small number of patients and lack of information concerning prior therapy make any conclusion hazardous in this setting. The data for platinum, although anecdotal, is significant because these patients had advanced disease with extensive prior therapy.[40,41] Four of five patients receiving platinum as a single agent achieved a complete remission.

A variety of combination chemotherapy programs have been utilized in metastatic seminoma, and these are depicted in Table III. Again, with such small numbers, wide-sweeping generalizations are not justified. Nevertheless, I fail to see any date to indicate that our preference for platinum + vinblastine + bleomycin as first-line chemotherapy in nonseminomatous testicular cancer should not be equally applicable for metastatic seminoma, especially since platinum as a single agent produced four of five complete remissions and vin-

TABLE III.
Combination Chemotherapy in Seminoma

Drug Regimen[a]	No. Patients	CR	PR	Reference
VCR + MTX + L-PAM	3	1	2	42
VCR + MTX + CTX	1	0	1	42
ABO	1	0	1	43
VAB-I	2	0	0	44
VB-I	10	6	2	45–46

[a] Abbreviations: VCR = vincristine, MTX = methotrexate, L-PAM = melphalan, CTX = cyclophosphamide, ABO = adriamycin + bleomycin + vincristine, VAB-I = vinblastine + actinomycin-D + bleomycin, VB-I = vinblastine + intermittent bleomycin.

blastine + bleomycin combination chemotherapy achieved six complete and two partial remissions in 10 patients with metastatic seminoma.[45,46]

Platinum + Vinblastine + Bleomycin

In 1974, combination chemotherapy with platinum + vinblastine + bleomycin was instituted as first-line chemotherapy in disseminated testicular cancer at Indiana University.[47] Patients with disseminated seminoma were treated with the same drug regimen as nonseminomatous tumors, although the vinblastine dosage was frequently lowered because of extensive prior radiotherapy. All subsequent chemotherapy programs at Indiana University likewise combined seminomatous and nonseminomatous tumors. I could not find any rationale for the use of single-agent alkylating agent therapy, or the inclusion of alkylating agents as part of our combination chemotherapy protocol.

There were four patients with disseminated seminoma included in our original series of 47 patients treated with platinum + vinblastine + bleomycin. All patients had extensive prior radiotherapy except for one patient who had a large Stage II anaplastic seminoma with an elevated HCG. This patient was treated initially with orchiectomy plus retroperitoneal dissection, but was found to have unresectable disease at which time he was referred to Indiana University, following a debulking procedure. A complete remission was obtained with platinum + vinblastine + bleomycin, and he has remained continuously free of disease for 32 months. Perhaps similar success could have been obtained with radiotherapy, but because of his initial elevation of HCG and histology (anaplastic seminoma) it was opted to treat him with chemotherapy instead. The probability of inducing a complete remission with platinum + vinblastine + bleomycin in patients with minimal metastatic disease and no prior chemotherapy or radiotherapy has been 98% in our experience (49 of 50 patients), and only three of these patients (6%) have ever relapsed. Since I do not feel the chemosensitivity of seminoma differs from the nonseminomatous tumors, I still feel that therapeutic approach to be preferable for similar patients.

The other three patients in our original series all had prior radiotherapy. One of these patients has a primary retroperitoneal seminoma, and received extensive abdominal radiotherapy on two separate occasions, as well as previous chlorambucil (no response). He was seen initially at Indiana University during his third relapse, with advanced hepatic, abdominal, and pulmonary metastases. Despite a 50% dosage reduction of vinblastine to 0.2 mg/kg, he experienced profound and prolonged myelosuppression. He achieved partial remission after two courses, but subsequent chemotherapy (including single-agent platinum) was given very irregularly because of prolonged thrombocytopenia and leukopenia. This patient relapsed after a 7-month partial remission and died shortly thereafter. Clearly, extensive prior radiotherapy (and chlorambucil) caused major delays in his chemotherapy, which may have played a role in his ultimate demise.

Another patient with pure seminoma was treated initially with radiotherapy for Stage II disease. He had four relapses over the ensuing 3 years, all treated (and locally controlled) with further radiotherapy. He also received chlorambucil, methotrexate, actinomycin-D, and vincristine during these time periods. He was initially evaluated at Indiana University in 1976, at which time he had massive ascites, hepatic, pulmonary, and nodal metastases. Although a brief partial remission (4 months) was attained, he subsequently relapsed and died of metastatic seminoma.

The last patient in this series has previously been reported.[20] He underwent an orchiectomy in 1974 which revealed pure seminoma, and had a positive lymphangiogram and normal lung tomograms. Because he had a significantly elevated HCG, he underwent a bilateral retroperitoneal lymphadenectomy (rather than radiotherapy), at which time all gross disease was removed, and his HCG fell to normal. Because histologically he had 13 positive nodes for metastatic seminoma (no other cell elements seen in any nodes), he received postoperative radiotherapy to the retroperitoneum, mediastinum, and left supraclavicular fossa. However, several months later he developed bilateral pulmonary metastases and his HCG again rose. A rapid, complete remission was achieved, although he also had severe and prolonged myelosuppression. A further complication was recurrent small bowel obstruction. This has been previously described in patients with prior abdominal radiotherapy receiving vinblastine.[48] Because of this, he only received 3 months of maintenance therapy with vinblastine, and then all chemotherapy was discontinued. Four months later, he was admitted to our Veterans' Administration Hospital with klebsiella pneumonia. At that time, his granulocyte count had returned to normal and he had been off all therapy for 3 months. Despite antibiotics and vigorous supportive care, he eventually died of his pneumonia. This patient was a chronic alcoholic and that may have been a predisposing factor. At autopsy, there was no gross or microscopic evidence of tumor.

All three of these patients with prior extensive radiotherapy had severe and prolonged myelosuppression, despite initial dosage attenuation and further dose reduction, and delay in subsequent courses. Furthermore, there is a significantly higher incidence of small bowel damage from vinblastine in patients with prior radiotherapy,[48] and this was the case of major morbidity in one of our patients. Another potential serious problem in such patients is pulmonary fibrosis, because the radiotherapy field encompasses the mediastinum, and such prior radiotherapy increases the incidence of bleomycin-induced pulmonary fibrosis.[49]

Initially, we salvaged only one of four patients with metastatic seminoma, although two of four patients initially achieved a complete remission. In June 1976, we began a random prospective study to evaluate different dosages of vinblastine, with and without adriamycin (see chapter on management of disseminated testicular cancer). Once again, we did not separate disseminated seminoma from the other cell types. The patient populations from these two studies can be seen in Table IV, and the results of treatment in Table V.

The median age was 36 (range 16–45). This is 10 years older than the median

TABLE IV.

Patient Population

Patient	Age	Histology	Prior Therapy[a]	Metastatic sites
1	33	anaplastic	orchiectomy & RND	retroperitoneal nodes
2	30	seminoma	XRT; chlorambucil + methotrexate + actinomycin-D + vincristine	liver, lungs, nodes, ascites
3	45	seminoma	XRT; chlorambucil	liver, abdomen, nodes, lungs
4	45	seminoma	RND + XRT	lungs
5	41	seminoma	XRT	abdomen, nodes, bone
6	23	anaplastic	None	lungs, abdomen, nodes, bone
7	45	anaplastic	RND (tumor incompletely removed)	abdomen, nodes
8	16	anaplastic	None	liver, lungs, abdomen, nodes
9	33	anaplastic	RND	supraclavicular nodes
10	43	seminoma	XRT	brain, lungs
11	34	seminoma	XRT	elevated HCG & AFP only
12	38	seminoma	XRT	abdomen, nodes

[a] Abbreviations: RND = retroperitoneal node dissection, XRT = radiotherapy.

TABLE V.

Treatment Results

Patient	HCG[a]	AFP[b]	Response	Duration (months)	Survival (months)
1	N	N	CR	32+	33+
2	53	N	PR	4	5
3	86	N	PR	7	8
4	153	N	CR	9[c]	10
5	N	N	CR	28+	30+
6	N	N	CR	26+	28+
7	870	675	CR	12+	13+
8	N	N	PR	3	6
9	N	N	CR	15+	16+
10	1320	N	PR	6	18+
11	73	86	CR	24+	25+
12	20	N	CR	14+	15+

[a] N = Normal (less than 1.5 mIU/ml).
[b] N = Normal (less than 20 ng/ml).
[c] Died of Klebsiella pneumonia; no tumor at autopsy.

age of patients treated during the same time period with disseminated nonseminomatous germ cell tumors. The median follow-up was 28 months (range 13–33 months). Five patients (42%) had anaplastic seminoma and the other seven had "typical" seminoma. This is a considerably higher incidence of anaplastic seminoma than expected, but this is a skewed patient population presenting with Stage III or IV seminoma or relapsing after previous radiotherapy.

Seven patients (58%) had elevated serum HCG levels, and two patients also had elevated alphaptoprotein. These latter two patients probably had nonseminomatous elements in their metastatic lesions, and some of the patients with elevated HCG likewise probably no longer exhibited a "pure seminoma" histology in their metastatic lesions. The problem of the definition of "metastatic seminoma" in patients with elevated serum markers has previously been discussed in this chapter. Nevertheless, most comparable series of chemotherapy of metastatic seminoma did not have the availability of radioimmunoassy HCG and AFP, and all patients *pathologically* had pure seminoma in their initial presentation. It is noted that four of five patients with negative HCG and AFP achieved complete remission and remain alive and disease-free.

All patients received platinum 20 mg/M^2 for 5 consecutive days. Most patients had three or four courses. Bleomycin was given in a dosage of 30 units weekly. An attempt was made in all patients to give 12 weeks (360 units) of bleomycin, but prior mediastinal radiotherapy limited the total bleomycin dosage in several patients. Vinblastine was given in full dosage, initially, if no prior radiotherapy had been administered; otherwise, the initial dosage was reduced 25%. Many previously irradiated patients had further dosage reduction.

During the past 2½ years, we have had a minor philosophical change in our treatment strategy in patients with metastatic seminoma and prior radiotherapy. All courses are given on time, regardless of the level of myelosuppression at the next course. This treatment strategy is also employed in disseminated *nonseminomatous* germ cell patients with prior radiotherapy. It is fully expected that the second course of platinum + vinblastine + bleomycin will be given at a time when the granulocyte count may still be less than 1000/mm^3, and the hemoglobin and platelet counts likewise may be severely compromised. Obviously, such a therapeutic strategy requires vigorous supportive care if necessary. However, hyperalimentation, prophylactic antibiotics, and protected environments were not deemed necessary, and granulocyte transfusions were nearly required. Packed cell and platelet transfusions were frequently employed, and appropriate cultures and immediate antibiotic therapy with carbenicillin and cephalosporin was started in any patient with a temperature above 38.3° C and less than 1000 granulocytes/mm^3. Aminoglycosides should be avoided, if possible, in this clinical situation because of the possible synergistic renal tubular damage between platinum and aminoglycoside antibiotics.[50] This treatment regimen is depicted in Table VI. Ten patients were treated with platinum + vinblastine + bleomycin and two patients (nos. 7 and 11) also received adriamycin. No vinblastine dose reduction was made unless the patient required hospitalization for granulocy-

TABLE VI.

Remission Induction

1. Platinum 20 mg/M^2 X 5 days every 3 weeks for 4 courses
2. Vinblastine 0.3 mg/kg every 3 weeks for 4 courses
3. Bleomycin 30 units weekly for 12 weeks

topenic fever. After completion of remission induction therapy, most patients received maintenance vinblastine, usually at a dosage of 0.2 mg/kg every 4 weeks for a total of 2 years of chemotherapy. Since institution of this treatment policy of not delaying subsequent courses regardless of the present level of myelosuppression, six of eight patients (75%) achieved complete remission, and all six remain free of disease.

Overall, eight of 12 patients (67%) achieved complete remission. There were no relapses, but one patient died of klebsiella pneumonia while still in complete remission. Thus, seven of 12 (58%) remain alive and disease-free from 12+ to 32+ months. In all our previous chemotherapy experience with disseminated testicular cancer, those patients relapsing after a complete remission invariably did so within a year of initiation of chemotherapy.[47] These results in metastatic seminoma are quite comparable to the results in disseminated nonseminomatous tumors with platinum + vinblastine + bleomycin.

Four of five patients with no prior radiotherapy achieved complete remission. The only failure in this group was a patient with massive hepatic metastases. The toxicity in these five patients was considerably less than that seen in the seven patients with prior irradiation.

The major determinant for inducing a complete remission, once again, was extent of metastatic disease. All five patients with minimal metastatic disease (no pulmonary metastases larger than 2 cm in diameter and no palpable abdominal mass and no hepatic or brain metastases) achieved complete remission, and all five remain alive and disease-free. Only three of seven advanced presentations achieved a complete remission, and only two are currently alive and disease-free.

Conclusion

My personal philosophy for the management of seminoma has been discussed, and our results with platinum combination chemotherapy presented. At Indiana University, we make the following recommendations:

1. Clinical State I or II typical or anaplastic seminoma with negative HCG and AFP should be treated with appropriate radiotherapy alone.
2. All anaplastic seminomas with HCG above 20 mIU/ml and all Stage III anaplastic seminomas should be treated as "nonseminomatous tumors," i.e., retroperitoneal lymphadectomy for clinical Stage I or II (without postoperative and/or preoperative irradiation) and chemotherapy for Stage III.

3. All Stage III seminomas should be treated initially with chemotherapy.
4. Any type of seminoma with an elevated AFP should be managed as a nonseminomatous tumor.
5. Platinum + vinblastine + bleomycin should be first-line chemotherapy for metastatic seminoma whenever chemotherapy is indicated.
6. The role, if any, of alkylating agents in metastatic seminoma remains to be determined.

References

1. Mostofi, F. K.: Testicular tumors. Epidemiologic, etiologic and pathologic features. *Cancer* **32:**1186–1201, 1973.
2. Maier, J. G., Mittemyer, B. T., and Sulak, M. H.: Treatment and prognosis in seminoma of the testis. *J Urol* **99:**72–78, 1968.
3. Notter, G., and Ranudd, N. E.: Treatment of malignant testicular tumors. A report on 355 patients. *Acta Radiol Ther Phys Biol* **2:**273–301, 1964.
4. Maier, J. G., Sulak, M. H., and Mittemyer, B. T.: Seminoma of the testis: Analysis of treatment success and failure. *Am J Roentgenol* **102:**596–602, 1968.
5. Hussey, D. H., and Doornbos, J. F.: *Treatment: Radiation Therapy in Testicular Tumors.* Flushing, N. Y.: Medical Examination Publishing Company, 1976, pp. 181–203.
6. Quivey, J. M., Fu, K. K., Herzog, K. A., Weiss, J. M., and Phillips, T. L.: Malignant tumors of the testis: Analysis of treatment results and sites and causes of failure. *Cancer* **39:** 1247–1253, 1977.
7. Maier, J. G., and VanBuskirk, K.: Treatment of testicular germ cell malignancies. *J Am Med Assoc* **213:**97–98, 1970.
8. Cionini, L., Ciatto, S., Pirtoli, L., Santoni, R., and Cappellini, M.: Radiotherapy of seminoma of the testis. Report on 129 patients. *Tumori* **64:**183–192, 1978.
9. Freedman, M. and Purkayastha, M. C.: Recurrent seminoma: Management of late metastases and recurrence of a second primary tumor. *Am J Roentgenol Radium Ther Nucl Med* **83:**25–42, 1960.
10. Kademian, M., Bosch, A., Caldwell, W. L., and Jaeschke, W.: Anaplastic seminoma. *Cancer* **40:**3082–3086, 1977.
11. Johnson, D. E., Gomez, J. J., and Ayala, A.: Anaplastic seminoma. *J Urol* **114:**80–82, 1975.
12. Lamm, D. L., Wepsic, H. T., Feldman, P., *et al.*: Importance of alphafetoprotein in patients with seminoma. *Urology* **10:**233–237, 1977.
13. Teilum, G., Albrechtsen, R., and Norgaard-Pedersen, B.: Immunofluorescent localization of alphafetoprotein synthesis in endodermal sinus tumor (yolk-sac tumor). *Acta Pathol Microbiol Scand (A)* **82:**586–593, 1974.
14. Nochomovitz, L. E., and Rosai, J.: Current concepts on the histogenesis, pathology and immunochemistry of germ cell tumors of the testis. *Sommer's Pathology Annual*, Part 1, #13, 1978.
15. Javadpour, N., McIntire, K. R., Waldmann, T. A., and Bergman, S. M.: The role of alphafetoprotein and human chorionic gonadotropin in seminoma. *J Urol* **120:**687–690, 1978.
16. Lange, P. H., McIntire, K. R., Waldmann, T. A., Hakala, T. R., and Fraley, E. E.: Alphafetoprotein and human chorionic gonadotropin in the management of testicular tumors. *J Urol* **118:**593–596, 1976.
17. Cochran, J. S.: The seminoma decoy: Measurement of serum human chorionic gonadotropin in patients with seminoma. *J Urol* **116:**465–466, 1976.

18. Mostofi, F. K., and Price, E. B.: Tumors of the male genital system *Atlas of Tumor Pathology,* 2nd Series, Fasc. 8. Washington, D. C.: Armed Forces Institute of Pathology, 1973, p. 38.

19. Braunstein, G. D., Vaitukaitis, J. L., Carbone, P. P., *et al.*: Ectopic production of human chorionic gonadotropin by neoplasms. *Ann Intern Med* **78:**39–45, 1974.

20. Lange, P. H., Nochomovitz, L. E., Rosai, J., Fraley, E. E., and The Seminoma Study Group: Serum alphafetoprotein and human chorionic gonadotropin in patients with seminoma: Analysis of 31 cases. Manuscript submitted to *J Urol,* 1979.

21. Peckham, M. J., and McElwain, T. J.: Radiotherapy of testicular tumors. *Proc R Soc Med* **67:**300–303, 1974.

22. Chebotareva, L. I.: Late results of sarcolysin therapy in tumors of the testes. *Acta UN Int. Congr Cancer* **20:**380–381, 1964.

23. Blokhin, N., Larionov, L., Perevodchikova, N., Chebotareva, L. and Merkulova, N.: Classical experiences with sarcolysin in neoplastic diseases. *Ann NY Acad Sci* **68:**1128–1132, 1958.

24. Whitmore, W. F., Smith, A., Yagoda, A., Cvitkovic, S. T., and Golbey, R.: Chemotherapy of seminoma. *Recent Results Cancer Res* **60:**244–249, 1977.

25. MacKenzie, A. R.: Chemotherapy of metastatic testicular cancer: Results in 154 patients. *Cancer* **19:**1369–1376, 1966.

26. MacKenzie, A. R.: The chemotherapy of metastatic seminoma. *J Urol* **96:**790–793, 1966.

27. Buckner, C. D., Clift, R. A., Fefer, A., *et al.*: High dose cyclophosphamide (NSC-26271) for the treatment of metastatic testicular neoplasms. *Cancer Chemother Rep* **58:**709–714, 1974.

28. Allaire, F. J., Thieme, E. T., and Korst, D. R.: Cancer chemotherapy with 5-fluorouracil alone and in combination with x-ray therapy. *Cancer Chemother Rep* **14:**59–75, 1961.

29. Hyman, G. A., Ultmann, J. E., and Habif, D. V.: Factors to be considered in the clinical evaluation of a new chemotherapeutic agent (5-fluorouracil). *Cancer Chemother Rep* **16:**397–399, 1962.

30. Livingston, R. B., and Carter, S. K.: *Single Agents in Cancer Chemotherapy.* New York: IFI/Plenum Inc., 1970, pp. 271–278.

31. Wilson, W.: Chemotherapy of human solid tumors with 5-fluorouracil. *Cancer* **13:**1230–1239, 1960.

32. Warwick, O. H., Alison, R. E., and Darte, J. M.: Clinical experience with vinblastine sulfate. *Can Med Assoc J* **85:**579–583, 1961.

33. Samuels, M. L., and Howe, C. D.: Vinblastine in the management of testicular cancer. *Cancer* **25:**1009–1017, 1970.

34. Hill, G. T., Sedransk, N., Rochlin, D., *et al.*: Mithramycin (NSC24559) therapy of testicular tumors. *Cancer* **30:**900–908, 1972.

35. Kennedy, B. J.: Metabolic and toxic effects of mithramycin during tumor therapy. *Am J Med* **49:**494–503, 1970.

36. Kennedy, B. J.: Mithramycin therapy in advanced testicular neoplasms. *Cancer* **26:**755–766, 1970.

37. Spear, P. W.: Clinical trial with mithramycin. *Cancer Chemother Rep* **29:**109–110, 1963.

38. Pitts, N.: Clinical data accumulated by Pfizer for NDA for mithramycin. *Proceedings of the Chemotherapy Conference on Mithramycin.* Carter, S. K. and Friedman, M. (Eds.). Bethesda, Md.: Cancer Therapy and Evaluation Program, National Cancer Institute, 1970, pp. 33–44.

39. Bonadonna, G.: Chemotherapy of testicular tumors. *Acta Chir Belg* **4:**393–400, 1971.

40. Higby, D. F., Wallace, H. J., Albert, D. J., and Holland, J. F.: Diamminodichloroplatinum in the chemotherapy of testicular tumors. *J Urol* **112**:100–104, 1974.

41. Samuels, M. L., Lanzotti, V. J., Boyle, L. E., Holoye, P. Y., and Johnson, D. E.: An update of the velban-bleomycin program in testicular neoplasia with a note on cis-dichlorodiamminoplatinum. *Cancer Chemotherapy III.* New York: Grune and Stratton, 1978, pp. 195–203.

42. Solomon, J., Steinfeld, J. L., and Bateman, J. R.: Chemotherapy of germinal tumors. *Cancer* **20**:747–750, 1967.

43. Burgess, M. A., Einhorn, L. H., and Gottlieb, J. A.: Treatment of metastatic germ cell tumors in males with adriamycin plus vincristine plus bleomycin. *Cancer Treat Rep* **61**:1447–1451, 1977.

44. Wittes, R. E., Yagoda, A., Silvay, D., McGill, G. B., Whitmore, W., Krakoff, I. H., and Golbey, R. B.: Chemotherapy of germ cell tumors of the testis. Induction of remissions with vinblastine plus actinomycin-D plus bleomycin. *Cancer* **37**:637–645, 1976.

45. Spiegel, S. C., Stephens, R. L., Haas, C. D., Jones, S. E., Lehane, D., Moon, T. E., and Coltman, C. A.: Chemotherapy of disseminated germinal tumors of the testis—comparison of velban-bleomycin with vincristine plus bleomycin plus actinomycin-D. *Cancer Treat Rep* **62**:129–130, 1978.

46. Samuels, M. L.: Treatment: Chemotherapy of testicular tumors. *Testicular Tumors.* Flushing, N. Y.: Medical Examination Publishing Co., 1976, pp. 204–223.

47. Einhorn, L. H., and Donohue, J.: Cis-diamminodichloroplatinum vinblastine and bleomycin combination chemotherapy in disseminated testicular cancer. *Ann Intern Med* **87**:293–298, 1977.

48. Samuels, M. L., Lanzotti, V. J., and Holoye, P. Y.: Radiation bowel injury complication velban-bleomycin stage III therapy of testis cancer. *Proc Am Soc Clin Oncol* **17**:266, 1976.

49. Einhorn, L. H., Krause, M., Hornback, N., *et al.*: Enhanced pulmonary toxicity with bleomycin and radiotherapy in oat cell lung cancer. *Cancer* **37**:2414–2416, 1976.

50. Dentino, M., Luft, F. C., Yum, M. N., Williams, S. D., and Einhorn, L. H.: Long-term effect of cis-diamminodichloroplatinum (CDDP) on renal function and structure in man. *Cancer* **41**:1274–1281, 1978.

8

VP-16-213: An Active Drug in Germinal Neoplasms*

Stephen D. Williams, M.D. and Lawrence H. Einhorn, M.D.

Department of Medicine, Indiana University Medical Center and Indianapolis Veteran's Administration Hospital, Indianapolis, Indiana

DRAMATIC IMPROVEMENTS in the therapy of disseminated germinal neoplasms have been made in recent years.[3,7] Testicular cancer, even in advanced stages, is now a highly curable disease. Of the initial 50 patients treated at Indiana University with the combination of cis-diamminedichloroplatinum (DDP) + vinblastine (Vlb) + bleomycin, 28 are now disease-free from 29 to 54 months.

An occasional partial responder will experience long survival.[4] However, in general, patients not rendered disease-free do poorly, with survival measured in months. In addition, in our experience about 15% of complete responders will relapse. Reinduction chemotherapy may yield a second complete response (CR); but unfortunately these are short-lived, and we have not seen long survival in this situation.

Another difficult patient population are those treated initially with Vlb + bleomycin and progress on this therapy. Previously, at our institution, such patients were treated with DDP + adriamycin (ADR). In 10 patients so treated, there was only one CR and no long-term survivors.[5]

The investigational epipodophyllotoxin VP-16-213 has been evaluated in a variety of hematologic malignancies and solid tumors.[6] It is among the most active agents in small cell lung cancer.[1] Its major dose-limiting toxicity is myelosup-

* Supported in part by Public Health Service, Grant #M01 RROO 750-06, and American Cancer Society Clinical Fellowship CF3678.

pression, which tends to be modest, and thus VP-16 appears to be suitable for combination chemotherapy. In addition, because its mode of action appears to be that of a spindle poison inducing a pre-mitotic block,[9] it theoretically could be synergistic with bleomycin.

Experience with this agent in germinal neoplasms is limited but promising. Table I summarizes available single-agent data.

Accordingly, this agent was evaluated either alone or in combination in patients with refractory germinal neoplasms.

Materials and Methods

Twenty-eight patients were treated with VP-16 alone or in combination. All had prior chemotherapy. The patient population is shown in Table II. Their ages ranged from 16 to 49. Five had primary extragonadal tumors. Three patients had seminoma and two choriocarcinoma. The remainder had embryonal carcinoma, teratocarcinoma, or mixed cell populations.

Several treatment regimens were used depending on the clinical situation. Group I consisted of two patients who had massive prior chemotherapy and were refractory to multiple standard agents including DDP and Vlb. They received VP-16 as a single agent.

The 17 Group II patients were treated with DDP + ADR + VP-16 ± bleomycin. All but one had received prior combination chemotherapy with either Vlb + bleomycin or DDP + Vlb + bleomycin. Eleven patients had shown clearly progressive disease while receiving Vlb and four other had attained only stable partial remissions (PR) on previous induction therapy. Several patients were also refractory to other agents.

The nine Group III patients received DDP + VP-16 ± bleomycin. All of these patients had received prior intensive combination chemotherapy, and six had previously progressed on Vlb.

Pretreatment evaluation included routine laboratory studies, chest x-ray, serum beta-subunit HCG, and alpha-fetoprotein by radioimmunoassay, and pulmonary function testing. Most patients had chest tomograms, abdominal ultrasonography, and computerized tomography.

Table I.
VP-16 in Testicular Cancer

Number of patients	Number of responses	Institution	Reference
5	4	Cambridge	8
a	1	Mayo Clinic	2
b	1	CALGB	2
4	1	EORTC	6

[a] Broad Phase II study with 1 of 20 responses; the only response was in a patient with testicular cancer.
[b] "1 of 16 responses in testis and ovary"; the response was in testicular cancer.

TABLE II.

Patient Population, Prior Therapy, Response, Duration

	Patient	Primary site	Histology	Prior therapy[a]	Response[b]	Duration (months)
Group I	1	testis	teratocarcinoma	surgery, RT Vlb + bleo DDP + Vlb DDP + ADR	PR	6
	2	extragonadal	embryonal	VAB-2 DDP + Vlb + bleo	PR	5
Group II	3	extragonadal	embryonal	DDP + Vlb + bleo HD MTX	PR	5
	4	testis	teratocarcinoma	DDP + Vlb + bleo	PR	8+
	5	extragonadal	choriocarcinoma	Vlb + bleo DDP + Vlb + bleo	PR	5+
	6	testis	embryonal	surgery RT Vlb + bleo	CR	13.5+
	7	testis	teratoma	DDP + Vlb + bleo	PR (NED after surgery)	8.5+
	8	testis	embryonal	surgery Vlb + bleo	CR	8.5+
	9	testis	embryonal	DDP + Vlb + ADR + bleo	None	
	10	testis	embryonal	surgery DDP + Vlb + Bleo	PR	5
	11	extragonadal	embryonal	surgery DDP + Vlb + bleo	PR (NED after surgery)	7+
	12	testis	embryonal	DDP + Vlb + bleo	PR	5+
	13	testis	embryonal	Act-D	CR	4+

TABLE II. *Continued*

Patient	Primary site	Histology	Prior therapy[a]	Response[b]	Duration (months)
14	testis	embryonal	DDP + Vlb + bleo Act-D Vlb	CR	4.5+
15	testis	teratocarcinoma	DDP + Vlb + bleo Act-D, chlorambucil	PR	4+
16	testis	seminoma	RT DDP + Vlb + bleo	None	3.5
17	testis	teratocarcinoma	surgery DDP + Vlb + bleo	PR (NED after surgery)	3.5
18	testis	embryonal	DDP + Vlb + bleo	CR	4+
19	testis	choriocarcinoma	surgery DDP + Vlb + bleo	CR	2+
Group III					
20	testis	teratocarcinoma	surgery, RT Act-D, CTX, Vlb + bleo DDP + ADR	PR	4
21	testis	teratocarcinoma	surgery, Act-D ADR + Belo + VCR DDP + Vlb + Bleo DDP + ICRF	CR	10+
22	testis	embryonal	COMF DDP + Vlb + bleo DDP + ADR + VCR + Bleo	CR	14+
23	testis	embryonal	DDP + Vlb + Bleo DDP + ADR + VCR + Bleo	PR	6+

24	testis	seminoma	RT DDP + Vlb + bleo	early death	
25	testis	embryonal	surgery, RT VLB + bleo	PR (NED after surgery)	4+
26	testis	embryonal	ADR DDP + Vlb + bleo	PR	2.5+
27	extragonadal	seminoma	surgery, RT CTX + VCR + 5-FU	CR	3.5+
28	testis	teratocarcinoma	surgery DDP + Vlb + ADR + bleo DDP + ICRF	CR	10+

a RT = radiotherapy; DDP = cis-platinum; Vlb = vinblastine; bleo = bleomycin; ADR = Adriamycin; Act-D = actinomycin-D; HD MTX = high-dose methotrexate; VCR = vincristine; CTX = cyclophosphamide; COMF = cyclophosphamide + vincristine + methotrexate + 5-flucrouracil.
b CR = complete response; PR = partial response; NED = no evidence of disease.

Induction therapy was given every 3 weeks for three to four courses. Drug dosages are shown in Table III. Every attempt was made to give all therapy on schedule regardless of degree of myelosuppression. VP-16 was given for 3–5 days depending on the patients expected hematologic tolerance.

Only two patients did not have prior exposure to bleomycin. Careful monitoring for bleomycin pulmonary toxicity was mandatory, and this agent was discontinued promptly in the presence of unexplained rales or a lag of expansion of a hemithorax on physical examination. An attempt was made however to complete an additional 12 weeks of bleomycin therapy (360 units).

During therapy with DDP, all patients received intravenous hydration with normal saline at 100 cc/hr, but mannitol and diuretics were not used.

If a course of therapy was followed by an episode of granulocytopenic fever, subsequent dosages of meylosuppression agents (ADR, VP-16) were reduced by 25%.

Complete remission was defined as normal serum markers, chest tomograms, and abdominal studies. Partial remission was defined as a 50% decrease in measurable tumor.

Results

Toxicity

As expected in this heavily pretreated patient population, toxicity was considerable during induction therapy. All patients had alopecia, nausea, and

TABLE III.
Treatment Regimens

Group I

VP-16 100 mg/M^2 over 30 min daily for 3–5 days[a] every 3 weeks until progression

Group II

Induction: Same VP-16
DDP 20 mg/M^2 IV over 30 min for 5 days every 3 weeks for 3–4 courses with continuous IV hydration
ADR 40-50 mg/M^{2*} IV push every 3 weeks for 3–4 courses
Bleomycin 30 units IV push weekly for 12 weeks (not given in one patient)[b]
Maintenance: VP-16 300 mg/M^2 IV over 1–2 hr every 4 weeks for 3 courses

Group III

Induction: Same VP-16
DDP 20 mg/M^2 IV over 30 min for 5 days every 3 weeks for 3–4 courses with continuous IV hydration
Bleomycin 30 units IV push weekly for 12 weeks (not given in four patients)[b]
Maintenance: VP-16 300 mg/M^2 over 1–2 hr every 4 weeks for 3 courses

---

[a] Depending on patients expected hematologic tolerance.
[b] These patients had previously progressed on this drug.

vomiting. Hematologic toxicity was marked. WBC nadir was 1100 cells/mm^2, platelet nadir was 60,000. Eight patients required hospitalization for leukopenia and fever, and four patients had documented infection. All of these episodes resolved, however, with appropriate management. Several patients required transfusion.

Two patients developed symptomatic nonfatal bleomycin-induced pulmonary fibrosis, and another developed abnormal liver function studies possibly related to VP-16.

Maintenance therapy was well-tolerated with mold nausea and modest hematologic toxicity.

There were no episodes of thrombocytopenic bleeding, clinically significant renal disease, or drug-related deaths.

Therapeutic Response

Response to therapy is summarized in Table IV. Both patients treated with VP-16 alone had PR's. Of the Group II patients, there were 6 CR's (35.3%) and 9 PR's (52.9%) for an overall response of 88.2%. Four of the PR's were rendered free of disease (NED) by resection of residual tumor (two mature teratoma; two residual carcinoma). Thus, 10 patients (58.8%) attained disease-free status. Of these, eight remain NED from 2+ − 13.5+ months (median = 5+ months). The likelihood of attaining disease-free status appeared unrelated to response to prior therapy.

There were eight evaluable Group III patients and one early death due to disease. There were 4 CR's and 4 PR's, one of whom underwent surgical resection of residual disease (mature teratoma). All five patients remain NED at 3.5+, 4+, 10+, 10+, and 14+ months.

Thus, of the entire patient population, there were 10 CR's (37.0%) and 15 PR's (55.6%). Another five patients had surgical resection of residual disease. Of the 15 patients attaining disease-free status, two have relapsed and 13 of 27 (48.1%) remain NED. Another nine patients are alive with disease.

Although the numbers are small, there was no obvious relationship between either pathology or primary site and response to therapy.

TABLE IV.
Therapeutic Response—Summary

	Patients	CR	PR	Early death	Progression
Group I	2	0	2	0	0
Group II	17	6	9	0	2
Group III	9	4	4	1	0
Total	28	10	15[a]	1	2

[a] Five subsequently had surgical resection of residual disease.

Discussion

Available Phase II data plus our two patients treated with VP-16 alone provide evidence that this agent has major activity in germinal neoplasms. To our knowledge, this is the only drug ever to induce objective response in patients refractory to DDP.

We believe that this study has defined several situations in which this drug is potentially useful. Very impressive is the fact that 23 of 25 patients responded to VP-16 combination chemotherapy and 15 ultimately attained disease-free status. It should be emphasized that this patient population was heavily pretreated, and all but two patients had received prior DDP-combination chemotherapy or Vlb + bleomycin. Many had progressed on Vlb. Previously, such patients at our institution were treated with DDP + ADR ± vincristine and bleomycin and, on occasion, investigational agents. However, complete responses were unusual, and long survival did not occur. Considered in this context, the results of this study are very impressive.

Length of follow-up in this study is relatively short. However, in our experience relapse from CR in vigorously restaged patients will occur in only 10–15%. Thus, we anticipate that a significant number of these patients will experience prolonged disease-free survival.

Thus, we believe VP-16 potentially useful in the following situations. First, this agent, in combination with DDP and ADR, should be considered for patients failing induction with Vlb + bleomycin.

Second, there are some patients treated with DDP + Vlb + bleomycin who only attain a partial response with residual unresectable disease. We currently give these patients maintenance Vlb and treat them immediately on progression with DDP + ADR + VP-16 + bleomycin. We prefer delaying further induction therapy until progression because this allows patients time to recover from toxicity of the prior regimen.

Third, a similar approach can be used for the occasional patient who relapses from a previous complete response while on maintenance therapy with vinblastine.

It should be emphasized that the regimens we use are very intensive with the potential for serious hematologic and other organ-system toxicity. However, toxicity is manageable if care is taken, and the approach should be aggressive as a realistic goal of such therapy is long-term disease-free survival and potential cure.

VP-16 has become an important component of combination regimens for patients with advanced refractory germinal neoplasms.

References

1. Cavalli, F., Sonntag, R. W., Jungi, F., et al: VP-16-213 monotherapy for remission induction of small cell lung cancer: a randomized trial using three dosage schedules. *Cancer Treat Rep* **62**:473–475, 1978.

2. Cancer Therapy Evaluation Program: Investigational Drug Branch annual report: VP-16-213. June, 1976.
3. Einhorn, L. H., and Donohue, J. P.: Cis-diamminedichloroplatinum, vinblastine, and bleomycin combination chemotherapy in disseminated testicular cancer. *Ann Intern Med* **87**:293–298, 1977.
4. Einhorn, L. H., and Donohue, J. P.: Combination chemotherapy in disseminated testicular cancer: the Indiana University experience. *Semin Oncol* **6**:87–93, 1979.
5. Einhorn, L. H., and Williams, S. D.: Combination chemotherapy with cis-dichlorodiammineplatinum (II) and adriamycin for testicular cancer refractory to vinblastine plus bleomycin. *Cancer Treat Rep* **62**:1351–1353, 1978.
6. EORTC, Clinical Screening Group: Epipodophyllotoxin VP 16213 in treatment of acute leukaemias, haematosarcomas, and solid tumors. *Br Med J* **3**:199–202, 1973.
7. Golbey, R. B., Reynolds, T. F., and Vugrin, Davor: Chemotherapy of metastatic germ cell tumors. *Semin Oncol* **6**:82–86, 1979.
8. Newlands, E. S., and Bagshawe, K. D.: Epipodophyllin derivative (VP-16-213) in malignant teratomas and choriocarcinomas. *Lancet:*9 July 1977.
9. Rozencweig, M., Von Hoff, D. D., Henney, J. E., and Muggia, F. M.: VM 26 and VP 16-213: a comparative analysis. *Cancer* **40**:334–342, 1977.

9

Brain Metastases in Testicular Cancer*

Stephen D. Williams, M. D. and Lawrence H. Einhorn, M. D.

Department of Medicine, Indiana University Medical Center and Indianapolis Veteran's Administration Hospital, Indianapolis, Indiana 46202

IN THE PAST 5 YEARS, significant advances have been made in the treatment of disseminated testicular cancer, with an increase in complete remission rate and survival.[1-3] The chemotherapeutic agents responsible for these advances, vinblastine, bleomycin, and cis-diamminedichloroplatinum, probably do not have active penetration through the "blood-brain barrier," although platinum is currently being evaluated by the Brain Tumor Study Group in glioblastomas. Because of the widespread hematogenous nature of germinal neoplasms, a propensity for brain metastases clearly exists. In other chemosensitive neoplasms, the central nervous system (CNS) has been a potential sanctuary for neoplastic growth. A primary example of this important clinical situation is childhood acute lymphoblastic leukemia, where successful remission induction therapy with prednisone plus vincristine improved the complete remission rate and survival.[4] Meningeal leukemia subsequently became "more common," presumably because more patients survived an adequate period of time to develop this complication of acute lymphoblastic leukemia. Prophylactic CNS therapy with cranial irradiation and intrathecal methotrexate has significantly prolonged survival.[5]

Small cell undifferentiated lung cancer is another neoplasm characterized by early and rapid hematogenous dissemination. Approximately 10% of these pa-

* Supported in part by Public Health Service Grant # M01 RROO 750-06 and American Cancer Society Clinical Fellowship CF 3678.

tients present with CNS metastases, and, at autopsy, 50% have evidence of CNS spread.[6] Recent advances with chemotherapy or chemotherapy plus radiotherapy in small cell lung cancer have produced higher remission rates, prolonged survivals, and improved the possibility of cure in this previously rapidly fatal disease.[7,8] However, the subsequent development of CNS metastases remains a potential barrier to curative therapy, and prophylactic cranial irradiation is now included in the treatment strategy of many of these patients.[6–8]

An important question in disseminated testicular cancer is whether some form of CNS prophylaxis should be employed in the management of these patients. The purpose of this paper is to determine that patient population developing CNS metastases, describe their clinical course and response to therapy, and determine if a subpopulation could be identified that might benefit from prophylactic CNS therapy.

Patient Population and Clinical Course

Between July 1973, and March 1978, 139 patients with disseminated germ cell neoplasms were treated with combination chemotherapy at Indiana University Hospitals. A variety of treatment regimens were used for these patients depending on the time period and therapy prior to referral to our institution.

Patients have symptoms or signs of central nervous system involvement had prompt radioisotope scans and frequently computerized tomography. Carefully selected patients with solitary lesions were considered for surgical resection and postoperative radiation therapy. Otherwise, whole brain irradiation alone was used. All patients received anticonvulsants, and steroids were used when indicated. Systemic therapy was continued as indicated.

TABLE I.
Patient Population

Chemotherapy regimen	No. patients	Follow-up (months)	CR	Alive	NED	Brain metastases (%)
ABO[a]	8	53–63	4	3	3	2 (25)
PVB[a]	50	22–46	33	33	28	5 (10)
PVB ± ADR[a]	59	4–21 (median = 11)	38	47	37	5 (8.5)
DDP + ADR[a]	10	4–26 (median = 8)	1	1	0	4 (40)
miscellaneous	12	2–16 (median = 7)	3	2	2	5 (42)
total	139					

[a] Abbreviations: ABO = adriamycin + bleomycin + oncovin (vincristine); PVB = platinum + vinblastine + bleomycin; DDP + ADR = platinum + adriamycin.

Table I outlines the patient population according to chemotherapy regimen, response, survival, and incidence of brain metastases. As can be seen, central nervous system spread was considerably more common in the platinum + adriamycin and miscellaneous groups. This was no doubt related to the fact that these groups were composed of heavily pretreated patients with far-advanced refractory disease.

Table II outlines the incidence of brain metastases related to cell type. Patients with yolk sac tumors and choriocarcinoma appear to have this complication more frequently.

Four patients had evidence of central nervous system involvement at the time of original diagnosis of metastatic disease, while an additional 17 patients developed this complication while on therapy. Two of these patients were in excellent partial remissions and still receiving platinum when the CNS lesions became evident. As expected, the four patients with involvement at diagnosis also had far-advanced systemic tumor. The median interval from diagnosis of testicular cancer until development of brain metastases was 18 months (range 0–9½ years). Median time from initiation of platinum combination chemotherapy to CNS spread was 6 months (range 0–19 months).

Presenting manifestations of CNS disease were as expected. All patients had symptoms or signs referrable to the central nervous system. Diagnosis was easily confirmed with radioisotope brain scan and/or computerized tomography. Twenty of our patients had such studies done (all positive), and compelling clinical evidence of brain metastases was considered sufficient in the remaining patient.

Table III shows the treatment given and survival according to treatment modality. Patients receiving no therapy were critically ill at the time of diagnosis and, as expected, had a very short survival.

TABLE II.
Incidence of Brain Metastases Related to Cell Type

Histology	Number	Brain metastases (%)
seminoma	11	2 (18.2)
choriocarcinoma	13	4 (30.8)
embryonal	69	7 (10.1)
teratoma	6	1 (16.7)
teratocarcinoma	34	4 (11.8)
yolk sac (testicular)	2	1 (50)
mediastinal yolk sac	4	2 (50)
total	139	21 (15.1)

TABLE III.

Treatment of Brain Metastases and Current Status

Treatment	Number	Dead	Survival from diagnosis of CNS spread
RT[a]	11	9	2-month median (range 1 week–21 + months)
surgery + RT[a]	3	3	5, 7, 11 months
none	7	7	2-week median (range 2 days–2 months)

[a] RT = radiation therapy.

Table IV reviews the clinical details of a subgroup of four patients who survived for at least six months free of clinically evident CNS disease. Two of these patients remain alive, although one has slowly progressing pulmonary metastases refractory to chemotherapy.

Analysis of cause of death reveals that only three patients were thought to die *exclusively* from CNS disease. Of these, one was moribund at diagnosis and received only supportive care. Another had CNS spread at first diagnosis of metastatic disease. He died from refractory CNS disease while in excellent peripheral remission. The third likewise died of recurrent CNS tumor after treatment with surgery and irradiation. He developed CNS disease several months after beginning chemotherapy. At death, he remained totally free of peripheral disease. Therefore, he is the only patient in this series who developed brain metastases after attaining durable chemotherapy-induced remission of peripheral disease and died exclusively of CNS tumor, and thus the only patient during this time period that would have derived possible benefit from prophylactic cranial irradiation.

Table IV.

Characteristics of Patients Surviving 6 Months Clinically Free of CNS Disease

Patient	Treatment	Histology	Survival (months)	Current status
1	RT[a]	Testicular yolk sac	21+	NED[b]
2	RT[a]	Seminoma	8+	alive with peripheral disease; CNS controlled
3	RT	Choriocarcinoma	6	Dead from peripheral disease
4	Surgery + RT	Mediastinal yolk sac	11	dead from peripheral disease

[a] RT = radiation therapy.
[b] NED = no evidence of disease.

Discussion

Brain metastases have been a relatively common event in our patients with disseminated germinal neoplasms, occurring in 15.1%.

CNS spread was a major cause of morbidity and mortality for our patients, as evidenced by a 1.5-month median survival from diagnosis. Currently available forms of therapy are inadequate.

We have defined certain subgroups of patients who appear to be at increased risk of developing CNS disease, namely patients with choriocarcinoma or yolk sac histologies, extensive prior therapy, or "massive disease." Recently, we have begun obtaining routine brain scans on such patients during their initial evaluation, prior to initiation of chemotherapy, even though they have no symptoms or signs of CNS disease. Hopefully, this may allow us to discover CNS metastases at an earlier time. Hopefully, the earlier diagnosis of CNS spread will lead to improved therapy for such patients. Likewise, determination of human chorionic gonadotropin in cerebrospinal fluid may prove useful in the diagnosis and monitoring of therapy, as it has in patients with gestational trophoblastic disease.[9]

Optimal therapy for patients with brain metastases remains unclear. Of interest, three of four patients who had 6-month or greater survivals after therapy had either yolk sac or seminoma histologies, usually more radiosensitive than other germinal neoplasms.

Although overall survival is very poor, enough patients had a sufficient quality and quantity of subsequent survival that, in our opinion, an aggressive therapeutic approach is warranted for most. This would include systemic chemotherapy when appropriate in addition to therapy directed at the CNS lesion.

The fact that two of our patients developed CNS disease while still responding systemically to platinum chemotherapy implies that clinically significant quantities of drugs employed did not penetrate the CNS. The utility of drugs known to cross the blood-brain barrier (i.e. nitrosoureas, VM-26, etc.) remains open to question.

It should be noted that there is experimental evidence that suggests that steroids may interfere with the antitumor action of DDP.[10] Consequently, we feel that steroids should not be used indiscriminately in patients receiving this agent.

Of the 17 patients who developed CNS spread subsequent to first diagnosis of metastatic disease, only two remained in durable systemic remission. One of these patients remains free of all disease, and the other died exclusively of CNS disease. Thus, ultimate curability could have been affected favorably by prophylactic central nervous system treatment in only one of 139 patients. Obviously, CNS prophylaxis is by no means known to be effective in this situation, and, thus, we have failed to identify a subgroup of patients who might benefit from this treatment.

Brain metastases are a late event in the natural history of germinal neoplasms, occurring in patients with advanced refractory disease. They are a major cause of morbidity and mortality, but occur in patients with active systemic tumor and thus only rarely affect ultimate survival. Current modes of therapy are inadequate, and surgical removal of solitary metastases is not clearly beneficial. As most of our patients with CNS spread had extensive chemotherapy prior to referral, it would appear that the best method of dealing with CNS disease is prevention by the application of the most effective systemic therapy possible early in the course of metastatic disease.

References

1. Samuels, M. L., Lanzotti, V. U., Holoye, P. Y., *et al.*: Combination chemotherapy of germinal cell tumors. *Cancer Treat Rev* 3:185–204, 1976.

2. Cvitkovic, E., Cheng, E., Whitmore, W. F., and Golbey, R. B.: Germ-cell tumor chemotherapy update. *Proc Am Soc Clin Oncol* 18:324, 1977 (abstract).

3. Einhorn, L. H., and Donohue, J.: Cis-diamminedichloroplatinum, vinblastine, and bleomycin combination chemotherapy in disseminated testicular cancer. *Ann Intern Med* 87:293–298, 1977.

4. Pinkel, D.: Five year followup of "total therapy" of childhood lymphocytic leukemia. *J Am Med Assoc* 216:648–658, 1971.

5. Simone, J., Aur, R. J. A., Hustu, H. O., and Pinkel, D.: "Total therapy" studies of acute lymphocytic leukemia in children. *Cancer* 30:1488–1494, 1972.

6. Bunn, P. A., Nugent, J. L., and Matthews, M. J.: Central nervous system metastases in small cell bronchogenic carcinoma. *Semin Oncol* 5:314–322, 1978.

7. Livingston, R. B.: Treatment of small cell carcinoma: evolution an future directions. *Semin Oncol* 5:299–308, 1978.

8. Einhorn, L. H., Bond, W. H., Hornback, N., and Joe, B. T.: Long-term results in combined modality treatment of small cell carcinoma of the lung. *Semin Oncol* 5:309–313, 1978.

9. Bagshawe, K. D., and Harland, D.: Immuno-diagnosis and monitoring of gonadotrophin-producing metastases in the central nervous system. *Cancer* 38:112–118, 1976.

10. Rosenberg, B.: Platinum coordination complexes in cancer chemotherapy. *Naturwissenschaften* 60:399–406, 1973.

10

Extragonadal Germ Cell Tumors *

Lawrence H. Einhorn, M.D.

Department of Medicine, Indiana University Medical Center and Veteran's Administration Hospital, Indianapolis, Indiana 46223

EXTRAGONADAL NEOPLASMS are among the most perplexing and embryologically intriguing entities in clinical oncology. These tumors are histologically identical to those of malignant germinal neoplasms of testicular origin, and can arise from the anterior mediastinum,[1-8] retroperitoneum,[6-13] or the pineal.[6,8,14] There are also isolated references to primary occurrences in such incongruous sites as the bladder,[15] prostate,[16] stomach,[17] and thymus.[5] Earlier authors usually hypothesized that these primary extragonadal tumors in reality arose from occult testicular primaries or represented dissemination after a spontaneous regression of a testicular primary.[12,13,18,19] It has only been in the last 15 years that firm evidence has been presented disputing these earlier theories and promulgating the existence of primary extragonadal neoplasms.[1-4,9,11]

The development of extragonadal tumors at these various sites is generally explained as the result of neoplastic transformation of primordial germ cells which have been displaced at various points along their normal pathway of migration to and from the urogenital ridge. Embryologically, the testes develop as an aggregation and maturation of primordial sex cells in and around the urogenital ridge, which early in embryologic development extends from the sixth cervical to the second sacral vertebra. From their site of origin in yolk sac endoderm, the

* Supported in part by PHS Grant M01 RR00 750-06.

primitive germ cells migrate along the dorsal mesentery of the hindgut to the urogenital ridge, and ultimately from there to the gonads. It is presumably along these pathways that occasional cells may become sequestered and under certain circumstances undergo neoplastic transformation. It is, of course, impossible to predict how many people develop such ectopic germinal epithelium. These germ cells are probably at a higher risk of developing malignant transformation, residing outside of the scrotum, for the same reasons that the undescended testis is prone to malignant degeneration.[20,21]

It is difficult to determine the exact incidence of extragonadal neoplasms. It is recorded in the British Tumor Registry that 1% of all patients with germ cell tumors had retroperitoneal tumors and palpably normal testes.[22] However, there are probably many patients with extragonadal tumors that go unrecognized by the pathologist and the clinician, and are labelled as a malignancy with an unknown primary. Some of these patients may be able to be diagnosed serologically (radioimmunoassay alphafetoprotein and beta subunit human chorionic gonadotropin) if not pathologically.[23]

There are several important concepts in the diagnosis and management of extragonadal neoplasm. First, these tumors should be treated in the same manner as their testicular counterparts, i.e., retroperitoneal or mediastinal seminomas should be treated primarily with radiotherapy, and extragonadal embryonal, teratocarcinoma, or choriocarcinoma should be treated with chemotherapy. Secondly, there is no indication for orchiectomy in these patients, unless the testis is abnormal to palpation. Lastly, and most important, this diagnosis must be considered in any young adult with an anterior mediastinal mass or retroperitoneal tumor which is pathologically interpreted as "malignant neoplasm—primary unknown." The proper diagnosis of this tumor representing a germinal neoplasm is critical because of the excellent prospects for cure with radiotherapy in mediastinal and retroperitoneal seminoma,[1,11] and the unique and potentially curative chemotherapy in nonseminomatous tumors.[24]

Abell[11] proposed that at least one of the following criteria be met for a diagnosis of retroperitoneal germinoma: (1) the presence of nonneoplastic gonadal tissue closely associated with the retroperitoneal lesion; (2) an encapsulated tumor without lymph node involvement; or (3) a high retroperitoneal neoplasm with adjacent lymph node involvement, but no involvement of the lower aortic, iliac, or pelvic lymph nodes. However, from a practical viewpoint, any retroperitoneal or mediastinal mass occurring in a patient without a detectable or subsequent appearance of a tumor in either testis and in whom the absence of metastatic disease in the lower aortic, iliac, or pelvic lymph nodes has been demonstrated should be considered as a primary extragonadal tumor if it meets the histologic criteria for such a malignancy.

This chapter will review the published series of extragonadal tumors as well as reviewing the experience with nonseminomatous extragonadal neoplasms treated with platinum combination chemotherapy at Indiana University. The nosology of these neoplasms lacked standardization, and, for the purpose of this paper only, the term "teratoma" will be used to describe a nonseminomatous tumor. Those extragonadal tumors seen at Indiana University were treated in the same manner as tumors arising in the testis, and, thus, many of these patients have been included in our previously published reports of chemotherapy in disseminated testicular cancer.[24,25] Endodermal sinus (yolk sac) tumors of the anterior mediastinum will be discussed separately at the end of this chapter.

Pathology

The histopathologic appearance of extragonad tumors is identical to the testicular counterpart. Extragonadal seminoma is a distinctive clinicopathologic entity. The uniformity of the tumor cells, the presence of a lymphoid infiltrate, with or without germinal centers, and the finding of epithelioid granulomas serve to distinguish seminoma from the more anaplastic teratomas and undifferentiated metastatic carcinomas. Epithelial or mesodermal structures can be seen in teratomas, and embryonal carcinoma can have elements of apparent adenocarcinoma. Syncytiotrophoblast and cytotrophoblasts in a plexiform pattern distinguishes choriocarcinoma. Also, gynecomastia, due to elevated beta subunit human chorionic gonadotropin (HCG), is most frequent with choriocarcinoma, and this finding should alert the clinician to the possibility of a teratoma (choriocarcinoma, embryonal, or teratocarcinoma).

The most frequent sites of metastases are the regional lymph nodes, lungs, liver, and bone. However, most of these tumors initially present as localized mediastinal or retroperitoneal masses. The high frequency of bone metastases[2,4] deserves emphasis since it is uncommon for testicular germinal tumors to spread to bone.[26] In those patients in whom distant metastases had occurred, the lesions were morphologically similar to the primary neoplasm.

Clinical Presentation and Behavior

The most frequent presenting symptoms for a primary mediastinal germ-cell tumor are chest pain, cough, and dyspnea. Less frequently, these tumors are diagnosed by a routine chest x-ray in an asymptomatic patient.

Abdominal pain or a palpable abdominal mass is the usual presentation of primary retroperitoneal germ cell tumors. These tumors, in either location, can attain a very large size, and this is probably the main reason why they behave more "aggressively" than their testicular counterparts. It is my impression that extragonadal neoplasms are not biologically different in their virulence or response to therapy then the same histological tumor arising in the testis; the poorer results, instead, are attributed to the larger volume of tumor at the time of presentation.

Primary Retroperitoneal Germinoma

Staemmler in 1934 was the first to observe ectopic testicular tissue within the retroperitoneum.[27] Unlike primary testicular tumors, the primary retroperitoneal germinoma will often reach enormous size before abdominal pain, back pain, anorexia, or weight loss are noted by the patient. The diagnosis is made at exploratory laparotomy, often to the surprise of the surgeon. As mentioned earlier, there is no clinical indication for orchiectomy in the patient with normal testes by palpation. Because of the difficulty eradicating very large retroperitoneal tumors with chemotherapy or radiotherapy, the primary retroperitoneal germinoma has a more ominous prognosis than do histologically identical tumors arising in the testis. However, primary testicular neoplasms with large retroperitoneal metastases probably have similar clinical behavior and responsiveness to therapy. It is important for the surgeon to be aware of this entity prior to exploratory lapartomy, and all reasonable attempts at surgical debulking should be attempted during the initial operation. There is no available clinical data indicating a therapeutic advantage for such surgical debulking, but it is a reasonable and realistic approach to pursue in an attempt to improve the prognosis in this patient population.

The choice of therapy and prognosis is dependent upon the histology. These tumors occur in the same age group and with the same histologic distribution as do primary testicular tumors, and similar therapeutic strategies should be employed. Retroperitoneal seminomas (pure seminoma with normal alpha-feto-protein and preferrably norml HCG as well) are best handled with radiotherapy, and have a considerably better prognosis than nonseminomatous tumors. Montague treated a patient with retroperitoneal seminoma with 3500 rad followed by chlorambucil, and the patient was still alive at 44+ months at the time of the publication.[10] Abell and co-workers reported on 10 retroperitoneal semi-nomas.[11] Seven were treated with radiotherapy, and three with surgery plus postoperative irradiation. Only three patients in that series died of neoplasm (5, 6, and 12 months). Another patient died from cardiovascular disease 13 years after radiotherapy, and had no evidence of seminoma at the time of his death. The other six patients remain alive at $\frac{1}{2}$, 2, 7, 16, 18, and 24 years. Johnson, *et al.* reported on the results of three retroperitoneal seminomas treated at M. D. Anderson; although all three patients died, the survival was 12, 30, and 47 months in this patient population.[6]

Overall, there were 14 retroperitoneal seminomas in these three series. Seven patients remain alive from 6 to 288 months, with four of those patients alive for 5+ years. An additional patient was a 13-year survivor, but died of unrelated causes. The median survival was 4+ years in these patients. These figures are comparable to those achieved with standard radiotherapy for Stage II testicular seminoma presenting with a large abdominal mass.[28]

Unfortunately, the prognosis for retroperitoneal teratomas was dismal. Montague treated four patients, and they all died of their tumor at 2, 8, 10, and

30 months.[10] These patients were all treated with Actinomycin-D and radio-therapy. The longest survival (2½ years) had a more indolent course, and survived long enough to receive three other chemotherapeutic trials (cytoxan + oncovin + methotrexate + 5-FU (COMF), mithramycin, and adriamycin). Utz and Buscemi reported on their experience with extragonadal tumors from 1950 to 1969 at the Mayo Clinic.[8] Unfortunately, this article did not delineate the patient population sufficiently well to ascertain individual outcomes. There were 12 mediastinal, five retroperitoneal, and one pineal body germ cell tumor. Eight of these were seminoma, and three were survivors for over 5 years. There were four long-term survivors (24+, 33+, 42, and 60+ months) in extragonadal tera-tomas. Unfortunately, the article does not state individual treatments, and it is not known whether any of these patients underwent complete surgical excision of his tumor. Johnson reported five patients with retroperitoneal teratomas.[6] The reported survivals were 3, 5, 6, 15, and 27 months respectively. Only the latter patient, a retroperitoneal choriocarcinoma, is still alive at 27+ months. Thus, combining all these series for retroperitoneal teratomas, the median survival was only 8 months, and was considerably worse than that reported for retroperitoneal seminoma.

A recent update of the M. D. Anderson experience for extragonadal germ cell tumors was presented by Luna.[29] Thirty-two patients (27 males) comprised the series which dated from 1944 to 1973. There were 13 mediastinal and 12 retro-peritoneal tumors. About half of these patients underwent autopsies, and the testes were carefully stepsectioned, and no evidence for a testicular primary was found. The mean survival was 12.4 months; only three patients survived beyond 4 years. These three patients all had extragonadal seminoma.

Primary Mediastinal Germinoma

The differential diagnosis of a patient with an anterior mediastinal mass should include lymphoma, germ-cell tumors, and thymoma. Germinomas account for 5–13% of all malignant mediastinal tumor.[30–32] Serum HCG and alphafetoprotein are useful diagnostic tools, and if a diagnosis of mediastinal germinoma is made, a routine "testicular cancer" workup should be undertaken, including careful palpation of testes, palpation for cervical or axillary lymphadenopathy, palpation of liver and liver function tests, lung tomograms, and abdominal ultrasound and computerized axial tomography. The majority of these patients will have disease initially localized in the mediastinum. The prognosis is considerably better for a mediastinal seminoma than for mediastinal teratomas.

Luna reported on 20 cases of mediastinal germ-cell tumors undergoing autopsy at M. D. Anderson from 1944 to 1975.[4] The mean age was 32.5 years, and the median survival was 10.9 months. There were only three survivors beyond 2 years (25, 35, and 44 months); two were seminoma and the other was embryonal plus seminoma. Only one patient (embryonal carcinoma) had an occult testicular primary. The authors point out that metastases to the anterior mediastinum (especially in the absence of other evidence of disease) are extremely rare in primary testicular cancer, and there seems little doubt that these cases represented primary mediastinal germ-cell tumors.

A separate M. D. Anderson series included seven patients with mediastinal germinoma.[6] It is not apparent how many patients were duplicated in Luna's series. There were three mediastinal seminomas; one died at 11 months and the other two remain alive at 4+ and 64+ months. All four mediastinal teratomas died of their malignancy at 1, 4, 8, and 26 months respectively.

Martini and co-workers presented the Memorial Sloan-Kettering experience of 30 mediastinal germinomas treated from 1949 to 1971.[2] Twenty-one patients had disease limited to the mediastinum at presentation. Only one of 20 mediastinal teratomas (a mediastinal choriocarcinoma treated with radiotherapy plus actinomycin-D plus methotrexate plus chlorambucil) remains alive (17+ months). The other 19 patients had a median survival time of only 7 months (range 1–16 months). Twelve of these patients received 4000 rad in 4 weeks without any significant clinical benefit. Twenty patients (including three seminomas) received some form of chemotherapy, usually an alkylating agent. Five of 10 mediastinal seminomas survived 10+ years. Two were treated with surgery alone, and are alive 20 and 24 years from diagnosis. One interesting patient initially treated with surgery plus radiotherapy was free of disease for over 10 years, but died of metastatic seminoma 12½ years after initial diagnosis. Four patients were treated with radiotherapy alone; one is alive and disease free at 12 years, one is alive but with active disease at 28 months, and two died (9 and 12 months from initiation of radiation). Three mediastinal seminomas in this series received chemotherapy plus radiotherapy: one is alive at 20 years and the other two died at 2½ and 3½ years from initiation of therapy.

Schantz and co-workers reported the Massachusetts General Hospital experience with mediastinal seminoma.[1] The mean age was 29.8 years. Sixteen of 21 patients are alive and well with a mean followup of 6 years. Five patients had surgery alone and except for one postop death (1 day after surgery), all are alive and well; 11 patients were treated with radiotherapy alone, and all are alive and disease-free. Only one patient presented with extrathoracic disease. Interestingly, this patient presented with anemia, fatigue, and cough, and was found to have a large mass that extended anteriorly to the sternum, posteriorly to the aortic arch, superiorly to the lung apices, and inferior to the pericardium. A subtotal resection was performed followed by 1500 rad. One year later, he developed bone metastases initially to the right femur and later to the left axilla, skull, cervical, and lumbar spine. All these areas were locally irradiated, and it is now 17½ years since the last known metastasis and he remains alive and free of disease. This extraordinary case exemplifies the radiocurability of seminoma, even when there is metastatic disease.

Cox presented the Walter Reed experience from 1949 to 1971 with mediastinal germinoma in his excellent paper.[3] Twenty-four patients were seen, and only five are still alive. Thirteen patients underwent autopsies, and, similar to the M.

D. Anderson experience, the testes were normal. Sixteen patients (67%) had tumor confined to the mediastinum. Nineteen patients were irradiated and only four received chemotherapy. Six patients had mediastinal seminoma. All six achieved complete remission with radiotherapy alone with no local recurrences, and four remain disease-free at 26, 27, 48, and 216 months. Two mediastinal seminomas died of pulmonary and osseous metastases after 4- and 28-month survivals.

Only one teratoma remains alive, a patient with embryonal carcinoma and seminoma treated with radiotherapy alone. He remains alive 19 years after initiation of radiation. Another patient with the same histology had a 7-year survival, but died of an acute myocardial infarction. The remaining 16 patients all died with a median survival of 5 months (range 1–9 months). Interestingly, six of eight patients with mediastinal embryonal carcinoma had permanent control of their primary with radiotherapy alone, but died of metastatic disease. The dosage employed was at least 4000 rad.

Cox also reviewed the literature on mediastinal germinomas. He found over 100 documented cases of mediastinal seminoma and concluded that 3000 rad in 3 weeks seemed sufficient to control this disease.[3] The radiocurability of mediastinal seminomas is well established. The experience with mediastinal teratoma has been considerably less encouraging. The median survival is less than a year, and the 5-year survival was under 10%.[3]

In summary, both retroperitoneal and mediastinal seminomas have an excellent cure rate (50–75%) with radiotherapy. It is interesting to note a significant cure rate with surgery alone as well. It is recommended that as much tumor should be removed as possible, followed by definitive radiotherapy. There does not appear to be an initial role for chemotherapy in extragonadal seminomas. The results for extragonad teratomas have been dismal with a median survival less than 1 year and less than 10% long-term survivors. It should be noted that most of these patients were treated with actinomycin-D and/or alkylating agents and usually with radiotherapy as well. These results are not dissimilar to those achieved with Stage III nonseminomatous testicular tumors in the 1960s with actinomycin-D. There does not appear to be a role for radiotherapy in the management of extragonadal teratomas, although the data from Cox with embryonal carcinoma is intriguing. In his series, there were two 5-year survivors with mediastinal embryonal carcinoma plus seminoma. It is also noteworthy that he achieved complete local control in six of eight mediastinal embryonal carcinomas with radiotherapy alone. Unfortunately, all these patients died within a year of diagnosis except for the two patients with embryonal carcinoma plus seminoma.

Since extragonadal tumors presumably should be treated in the same manner as their testicular counterparts, better results can be anticipated in these nonseminomatous tumors with modern aggressive chemotherapy. Samuels reported 21 patients treated with bleo-COMF or vinblastine + bleomycin.[33] There were five (24%) complete remissions, and all five remain alive and disease-free. There were seven partial remissions (33%), and the median survival time for all responders was 65 weeks and 47 weeks for the entire patient population.

Platinum Combination Chemotherapy

At Indiana University, extragonadal teratomas were treated in the same manner as disseminated testicular neoplasms.[24,25] Ten patients with extragonadal germ-cell tumors were treated with platinum combination chemotherapy from 1975 to 1978, and the patient characteristics are described in Table I. Nine of these patients were nonseminomatous extragonadal tumors (teratomas). The only seminoma was a patient with a primary retroperitoneal seminoma who was initially treated with surgery, radiation, and chlorambucil. Eight patients were treated with platinum + vinblastine + bleomycin, and two were treated with platinum + adriamycin.[25] These latter two patients had previously developed progressive disease during therapy with vinblastine plus bleomycin. The median age was 26 (range 18–53). Five patients had retroperitoneal primaries, and five had primary mediastinal tumors. The five patients with mediastinal teratomas all presented with chest pain, dyspnea, or cough, and were found to have a large anterior mediastinal mass on chest x-ray. These patients all required thoracotomy for diagnosis. Only one of these five patients had an attempt at debulking surgery; the other four patients had biopsy only. At the time of presentation, four of these patients had disease limited to the mediastinum. Four patients had elevated HCG, and two had elevated alpha-fetoprotein. The two patients treated with platinum + adriamycin had the most extensive disease, and both were acutely short of breath and required supplemental oxygen at the start of platinum combination chemotherapy. Both of these patients had significant objective and subjective improvement; but the duration of response was very brief (3 months each), and both patients died shortly after progressing on platinum plus adriamycin. The three patients treated with platinum + vinblastine + bleomycin all achieved complete remission, and all remain free of disease for 2, 13, and 24 months. The latter patient had over 90% of his tumor surgically excised prior to initiation of chemotherapy. We do not recommend mediastinal irradiation for these tumors, even though they are initially localized, as long-term survival with irradiation for mediastinal teratomas has been dismal. Furthermore, mediastinal irradiation can compromise subsequent bleomycin chemotherapy increasing the lung tissue susceptibility to pulmonary fibrosis.[34]

Five patients with retroperitoneal germinomas were treated with platinum combination chemotherapy. As mentioned previously, one of these patients had a retroperitoneal seminoma. Although this patient had initial control with radiotherapy, he later developed recurrent disease that failed to respond to chlorambucil. He had a 5-month partial remission with platinum + vinblastine + bleomycin, but subsequently progressed and died shortly thereafter. All five of these patients initially presented with abdominal pain and a huge abdominal mass. These patients were all diagnosed at laparotomy, and none of them had any initial attempt at surgical debulking. Two patients had primary retroperitoneal choriocarcinoma, and two had embryonal carcinoma. All five patients had elevated HCG at the initiation of platinum combination chemotherapy, and two had

TABLE I

Patient Population

Number	Primary	Prior therapy[a]	Therapy[b]	Area of tumor	Response	Duration (months)	Survival (months)
1	med. chorioCA	VB III	PH + ADR	mediastinum liver, cervical nodes	PR	3	5
2	med. embryonal	VB III; XRT	PH + ADR	mediastinum	PR	3	4
3	med. teratocarcinoma	none	PVB	mediastinum	CR	13+	14+
4	med. teratoma	surgery	PVB	mediastinum	CR	24+	24+
5	med. embryonal	none	PVB	mediastinum	CR	2+	2+
6	abd. chorioCA	ABO	PVB	liver, lung, bone	PR	4	7
7	abd. embryonal	none	PVB	liver, retroperito neum	NED with surg.	2	9
8	abd. seminoma	XRT + chlorambucil	PVB	retroperitoneum, lung, liver	PR	5	8
9	abd. embryonal	none	PVB	retroperitoneum and cervical nodes	NED with surg.	4+	9+
10	abd. chorioCA	none	PVB	retroperitoneum, liver, and lung	NED with surg.	18+	24+

[a] VB III = vinblastine plus continuous infusion bleomycin; XRT = mediastinal irradiation.
[b] PLT + ADR = platinum plus adriamycin; PVB = platinum plus vinblastine plus bleomycin.

concomitant elevation of alpha-fetoprotein. All five patients were treated with platinum + vinblastine + bleomycin, and none achieved a complete remission. However, three patients had a significant reduction in tumor mass, and a reexploration with complete removal of residual disease was accomplished (NED with surgery). All three of these patients had persistent carcinoma in the surgical specimen. One relapsed shortly after surgery, and the other two patients remain free of disease 4+ and 18+ months following surgical excision of residual disease. These results are comparable with our previously published results for primary testicular cancer with advanced abdominal disease.[24]

Five of these eight extragonadal patients treated with platinum + vinblastine + bleomycin remain alive and disease-free for 3, 9, 14, 24, and 24 months from initiation of chemotherapy. The other three patients died 7, 8, and 9 months after chemotherapy was started. Since our relapse rate has historically been 10–20% for patients achieving a disease-free status,[24] it is expected that most if not all of these five patients will remain disease-free. Although the numbers are small and the follow-up brief, there is a suggestion that these results will be significantly better than the previously reported series for extragonadal teratomas.

Yolk Sac Endodermal Carcinoma

The concept of endodermal sinus tumor (or yolk sac tumor) was introduced in oncology by the comparative studies of Teilum,[35] who presented a specific interpretation of the essential element in this tumor type in the ovary and testis. This tumor has a distinctive microscopic pattern with stellate cells forming a loose vacuolated network with wide meshes or a system of communicating cavities or channels.[36] Another characteristic feature is the occurrence of perivascular formations with mantles or starlike halos of cells of epithelial appearance and surrounded by capsular sinusold spaces.[36] This entity has been recogonized as a major component of testicular tumors of children, where it has a relatively favorable prognosis. It has only recently been recognized that many adult testicular tumors also contain yolk sac elements. Talerman studied 68 nonseminomatous adult germ-cell tumors of the testis and 26 (38%) had yolk sac elements.[37] Yolk sac was the predominant element in eight of these patients. There were no cases of pure yolk sac carcinoma of the adult testis in this series.

After the recognition of yolk sac tumors in the ovary and testis, similar tumors have been described in a number of extragonadal sites, including the anterior mediastinum.[38,39] It has also been shown that the so-called adenocarcinoma of the infantile testis is a yolk sac tumor mimicking the endodermal sinus structure.[40] It is important to realize that a primary mediastinal yolk sac tumor may also be misinterpreted as an adenocarcinoma.[23]

The normal yolk sac is one of the main sites of alpha-fetoprotein synthesis in the fetus.[41] The availability of a serum radioimmunoassay for alpha-fetoprotein has improved the diagnostic and therapeutic capabilities of the clinician. Patients with mediastinal yolk sac tumors should all have elevated serum alpha-fetoprotein which should disappear before a patient can be considered to be free of disease. Likewise, a relapse is often heralded by the reappearance of elevated alpha-fetoprotein levels.

Results of Therapy

Yolk sac carcinomas of the adult are rapidly progressing tumors. Ovarian yolk sac tumors are usually inoperable at diagnosis,[42] and survival has been dismal. However, recent reports of chemotherapy with vincristine + actinomycin-D + cyclophosphamide for ovarian yolk sac tumors look promising when used as a surgical adjuvant, and occasionally for inoperable lesions.[43] There are no similar reports of chemotherapy successes in mediastinal yolk sac tumors.

Primary mediastinal yolk sac tumors are among the most lethal malignancies in oncology,[38,39,44,45] and reports of survival beyond 1 year are exceedingly rare. Although this tumor is probably radiosensitive, there does not appear to be a beneficial effect upon survival with irradiation.

Results with Platinum

Many primary testicular tumors have yolk sac elements, and this may rarely be the predominant cell type.[37] In our initial series of 47 patients with germinal neoplasms treated with platinum + vinblastine + bleomycin, there were two testicular tumors that had as their predominant element yolk sac carcinoma.[24] Both of these patients have been disease-free and off all therapy for over 2 years.

Mediastinal yolk sac tumors have been the commonest form of primary germinal mediastinal tumors at Indiana University. Seven such patients have been treated with platinum + vinblastine + bleomycin from 1976 to 1978. All patients had elevated alpha-fetoprotein levels and normal HCG. The patients all presented with chest pain, dyspnea, and a larger anterior mediastinal mass, and all diagnosis were made at thoracotomy. Six of these patients were highly symptomatic with Karnofsky performance status of 60 or lower. The patient characteristics are depicted in Table II. Although the results were discouraging, nonetheless a significant antitumor effect was seen in all patients except for no. 3 (Table II). Most patients normalized their alpha-fetoprotein, but still had an abnormal chest x-ray. All patients had a 20–40 point improvement in their performance status, and most patients were asymptomatic after two courses of therapy. This was a remarkable achievement, since many of these patients were highly symptomatic at initiation of therapy.

Clearly, the optimal therapy for mediastinal yolk sac tumors has yet to be discovered. In all probability, it will require a combination of surgery plus chemotherapy and perhaps radiotherapy as well. Three typical patients with mediastinal yolk sac tumors treated at Indiana University are described below.

TABLE II

Patient Population Mediastinal Yolk Sac

Patient	Performance status	Extent of disease	Response		Duration (months)	Survival (months)
1	50	mediastinum	PR	3		8+
2	60	mediastinum	PR	4		7+
3	40	mediastinum and liver	none	—		2
4	60	mediastinum	PR	2		10
5	40	mediastinum and supraclavicular nodes	CR	2	(CNS relapse)	15
6	60	mediastinum	PR	4		8
7	80	mediastinum	PR	2+		3+

Patient No. 1: This patient is a 26-year-old male who presented to his referring physician with chest pain and dyspnea on exertion. A chest x-ray revealed a large anterior mediastinal mass. A thoracotomy was required for diagnosis, revealing a yolk sac endodermal carcinoma. At the time of admission for initiation of chemotherapy, he had an obvious superior vena caval syndrome, and a po_2 of

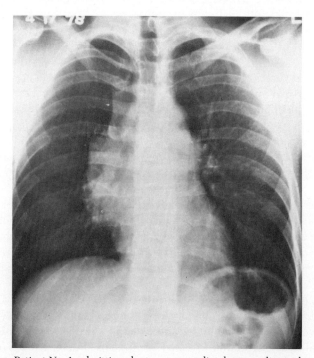

FIG 1. Patient No. 1: admitting chest x-ray revealing large mediastinal mass.

48. His initial chest x-ray is shown in Figure 1. His Karnofsky performance status (KPS) was 50. His admitting alpha-fetoprotein was 512 ng/ml. He also had an elevated lactic dehydrogenase (289) and alkaline phosphatase (234). He was started on chemotherapy with platinum + vinblastine + bleomycin on 4/17/78. After his first course of therapy, he became asymptomatic, did not require supplemental oxygen, and his alpha-fetoprotein decreased to 48. His chest x-ray was significantly improved. Following his second course of chemotherapy, his alpha-fetoprotein normalized, although his chest x-ray still revealed a persistent mediastinal mass. He received 4 full courses of platinum + vinblastine + bleomycin over a 12-week period. He then received a dosage of maintenance vinblastine (0.3 mg/kg intravenous push). He was readmitted 8/28/78 for evaluation of surgical resection of residual mediastinal disease. At that time, all studies were normal (including alpha-fetoprotein), except for his chest x-ray (Fig. 2), and he underwent a thoracotomy 9/1/78 with complete further resection of residual tumor. Histologically, this tumor was still yolk sac endodermal carcinoma. Because of the high likelihood for local recurrence, he was started on mediastinal radiotherapy 9/20/78. However, shortly thereafter, he developed recurrent pulmonary and mediastinal metastases (Fig. 3), and his alpha-fetoprotein rose precipitously to 2800 ng/ml. He was then started on VP-16 with further pro-

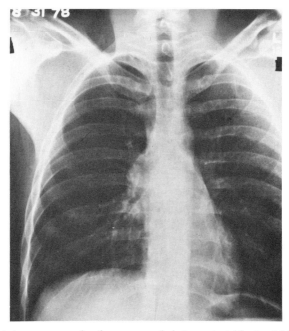

FIG. 2. Dramatic improvement after four courses of platinum + vinblastine + bleomycin; only small residual tumor remains.

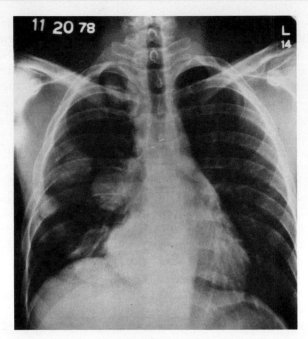

FIG 3. Rapid progression.

gression. He most recently has been on adriamycin + cyclophosphamide with further progression, and his last alpha-fetoprotein was 4860.

Comment: This patient presented acutely ill with a superior vena caval syndrome and had a partial remission with platinum plus vinblastine plus bleomycin. Because he was felt to be operable, a thoracotomy was done with complete removal of residual tumor. Despite normal alpha-fetoproteins, the resected tumor was persistent yolk sac carcinoma. Postoperative radiotherapy (at which time he was grossly free of disease) failed to prevent his subsequent rapid deterioration. A second partial remission has not been achieved with further chemotherapy. It is difficult to imagine any alternative therapeutic strategy that could have altered the ultimate outcome in this case.

Patient No. 10: This patient was a 33-year-old male who presented with sudden chest pain, cough, fever, and dyspnea. A thoracotomy revealed the diagnosis of yolk sac endodermal carcinoma, and he was transferred to Indiana University. His admitting chest x-ray at Indiana is shown in Figure 4. His alpha-fetoprotein was 1050 and on 10/3/77, he was started on platinum + vinblastine + bleomycin + adriamycin. He had an initial brief partial remission (Fig. 5), and his alpha-fetoprotein also normalized. However, his alpha-fetoprotein rose to 2000 on maintenance vinblastine, and, on 4/11/78, he was started on vincristine + actinomycin-D + cyclophosphamide (VAC) (Fig. 6). He developed further pro-

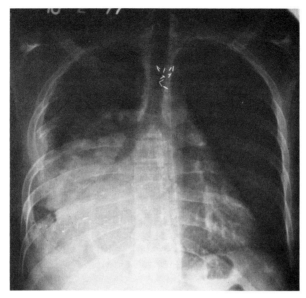

FIG. 4. Patient No. 4: admitting chest x-ray revealing massive disease.

gression, and, on 5/2/78, he was started on platinum + VP-16. He continued to rapidly deteriorate and he ultimately died on 6/3/78.

Comment: This patient also exhibited the fact that a normal alpha-fetoprotein

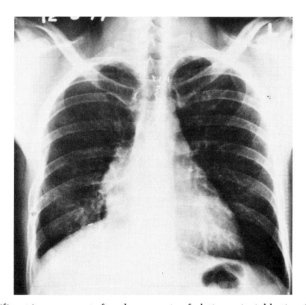

FIG. 5. Significant improvement after three courses of platinum + vinblastine + bleomycin.

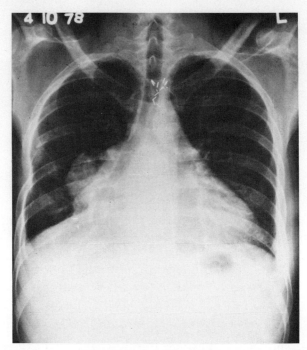

FIG. 6. Recurrent yolk sac tumor.

and a radiographical partial remission clearly does not imply eradication of viable tumor.

Patient No. 5: This patient was a 24-year-old male who presented with dyspnea, chest pain, and a large anterior mediastinal mass and supraclavicular lymphadenopathy. A node biopsy revealed yolk sac carcinoma, and he was referred to Indiana University. His admitting chest x-ray is shown in Figure 7, and his initial alpha-fetoprotein was 2600. This patient was acutely ill with a KPS of 40. He was started on platinum + vinblastine + bleomycin 1/10/77. After his first course, he had a dramatic subjective improvement, and an improvement objectively on his chest x-ray. He had further radiographic improvement after his second course (Fig. 8), and his alpha-fetoprotein became normal. He was given four courses (12 weeks) of platinum + vinblastine + bleomycin; a repeat chest x-ray and mediastinal tomograms were normal, and he was in a clinical complete remission and was started on maintenance vinblastine (0.3 mg/kg once a month). However, shortly afterwards, he developed a grand mal seizure, and was found to have a solitary brain metastasis which was completely removed at craniotomy on 6/7/77. He then received postoperative whole brain radiotherapy and two supplementary courses of platinum + vinblastine + bleomycin. However, he again developed progressive disease on 9/15/77 with increase in alpha-fetoprotein to 1760. At that time, his chest x-ray and brain scan were normal, and he was

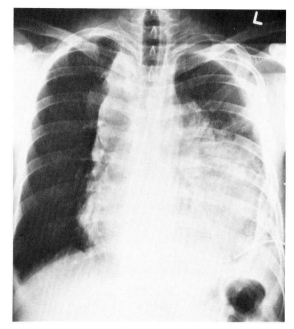

FIG. 7. Patient No. 7: admitting chest x-ray.

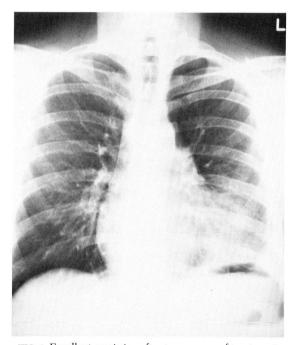

FIG. 8. Excellent remission after two courses of treatment.

started on vincristine + actinomycin-D + cyclophosphamide (VAC). Shortly thereafter, he developed new pulmonary nodules and was switched to adriamycin. He continued to have progressive disease, and he expired on 4/10/78.

Comment: This was the only complete remission in this series. Although his only initial relapse was in the brain, he later developed recurrent pulmonary disease.

Conclusions

1. Extragonadal germ cell tumors is a definitive clinicopathologic entity. There is no need to perform an orchiectomy on such patients.

2. The clinician and the pathologist need to be aware of this entity, especially in young males with a retroperitoneal or anterior mediastinal mass and an initial pathological diagnosis of "neoplasm—primary unknown."

3. These tumors should be treated in a parallel fashion to their testicular counterparts, and a similar evaluation and follow-up, including serum HCG and alpha-fetoprotein, should be performed.

4. Extragonadal seminomas have a high cure rate with radiation therapy.

5. Although previous results with extragonadal embryonal carcinoma, teratocarcinoma, and choriocarcinoma have been dismal, there is optimism that modern aggressive combination chemotherapy can improve the median survival and potential cure rate in these patients.

6. The results with mediastinal yolk sac tumors remain disappointing. Although meaningful remissions were seen with platinum combination chemotherapy, the survival was brief. New therapeutic strategies are needed in this tumor.

References

1. Schantz, A., Sewall, W., and Castleman, B.: Mediastinal germinoma. *Cancer* **30:**1189–1194, 1972.

2. Martini, N., Golbey, R. B., Hajdu, S. I., Whitmore, W. F., and Beattie, E. J.: Primary mediastinal germ cell tumors. *Cancer* **33:**763–769, 1974.

3. Cox, J. D.: Primary malignant germinal tumors of the mediastinum. *Cancer* **36:**1162–1168, 1975.

4. Luna, M. A., and Valenzuela-Tamariz, J.: Germ-cell tumors of mediastinum: Postmortem findings. *Am J Clin Pathol* **65:**450–454, 1976.

5. Schlumberger, H. G.: Teratoma of anterior mediastinum in group of military age—study of 16 cases and review of theories of genesis. *Arch Pathol* **41:**398–405, 1946.

6. Johnson, D. E., Laneri, J. P., Mountain, C. F., and Luna, M.: Extra-gonadal germ cell tumors. *Surgery* **73:**85–90, 1973.

7. Cha, E. M.: Ectopic seminoma in the retroperitoneum and mediastinum. *J Urol* **110:**47–53, 1973.

8. Utz, D. C., and Buscemi, M. F.: Extragonadal testicular tumors. *J Urol* **105:**271–274, 1971.

9. Das, S., Bochetto, J. R., and Alpert, L. I.: Primary retroperitoneal seminoma. *Cancer* **36:**595–598, 1975.

10. Montague, D. K.: Retroperitoneal germ cell tumors with no apparent testicular involvement. *J Urol* **113**:505–508, 1975.

11. Abell, M. R., Fayos, J. V., and Lampe, I.: Retroperitoneal germinomas (seminomas) without evidence of testicular involvement. *Cancer* **18**:273–290, 1965.

12. Friedman, N. B.: Comparative morphogenesis of extragenital and gonadal teratoid tumors. *Cancer* **4**:265–276, 1951.

13. Mears, E. M., Jr., and Briggs, E. M.: Occult seminoma of the testis masquerading as a primary extragonadal germinal neoplasm. *Cancer* **30**:300–306, 1972.

14. Simson, R. L., Lampe, I., and Abell, M. R.: Suprasellar germinomas. *Cancer* **22**:533–544, 1968.

15. Hyamn, A., and Leiter, H. E.: Extratesticular chorioepithelioma in male probable primary in urinary bladder. *J Mt Sinai Hosp* **10**:212–216, 1943.

16. Dvoracek, C.: Primary chorionepithelioma of prostate with gynecomastia. Cas Lek Cesk **88**:198–201, 1949.

17. Holt, L. P., Melcher, D. H., and Colquhoun, J.: Extragonadal choriocarcinoma in the male. *Postgrad Med J* **41**:134–141, 1965.

18. Rather, L. V., Gardiner, W. R., and Frerichs, J. B.: Regression and maturation of primary testicular tumors with progressive growth of metastases: a report of 6 new cases and a review of the literature. *Stanford Med Bull* **12**:12–24, 1954.

19. Azzopardi, J. G., and Hoffbrand, A. V.: Retrogression in testicular seminoma with viable metastases. *J Clin Pathol* **18**:135–141, 1965.

20. Campbell, H. E.: The incidence of malignant growth of the undescended testicle: a reply and re-evaluation. *J Urol* **81**:663–668, 1959.

21. Thurzo, R., and Pinter, J.: Cryptorchism and malignancy in men and animals. *Urol Int* **11**:216–231, 1961.

22. Collins, D. H., and Pugh, R. C. B.: Classification and frequency of testicular tumors. *Br J Urol Suppl* **36**:1, 1964.

23. Greco, F. A.: Personal communication.

24. Einhorn, L. H., and Donohue, J. P.: Cis-diamminedichloroplatinum vinblastine, and bleomycin combination chemotherapy in disseminated testicular cancer. *Ann Intern Med* **87**:293–298, 1977.

25. Einhorn, L. H., and Williams, S. D.: Combination chemotherapy with cis-diamminedichloroplatinum and adriamycin in testicular cancer refractory to vinblastine plus bleomycin. *Cancer Treat Rep* **62**:1351–1353, 1978.

26. Oberman, H. A., and Liboke, J. H.: Malignant germinal neoplasms of the mediastinum. *Cancer* **17**:498–507, 1964.

27. Staemmler, M.: Untersuchungen uber iiberzahlige Hodenanlagen in der Bauchhohle. *Verh Dtsch Ges Pathol* **27**:190, 1934.

28. Hussey, D. H., and Doornbos, J. F.: Treatment: Radiation therapy. *Testicular Tumors*, 2nd ed. Johnson, D. E. (Ed.). Flushing, N.Y.: Medical Examination Publishing Co., Inc., 1976, pp. 181–203.

29. Luna, M. A.: Extragonadal germ cell tumors. *Testicular Tumors*, 2nd ed. Johnson, D. E. (Ed.). Flushing, N.Y.: Medical Examination Publishing Co., Inc., 1976, pp. 261–265.

30. Joseph, W. L., Murray, J. F., and Mulder, D. G.: Mediastinal tumors—problems in diagnosis and treatment. *Dis Chest* **50**:150–160, 1966.

31. Conkle, D. M., and Adkins, R. B., Jr.: Primary malignant tumors of the mediastinum. *Am Thorac Surg* **14**:553–567, 1972.

32. Wychulis, A. R., Payne, W. S., Clagett, O. T., and Woolner, L. B.: Surgical treatment of mediastinal tumors. *J Thorac Cardiovasc Surg* **62**:379–391, 1971.

33. Samuels, M. L., Boyle, L. E., Nicholson, G. L., Smith, T., and Johnson, D. E.: Improved

survival of extragonadal germinal neoplasis with bleomycin combination chemotherapy programs. *Proc Am Assoc Cancer Res* **18**:147, 1977.

34. Einhorn, L. H., Krause, M., Hornback, N., and Furnas, B.: Enhanced pulmonary toxicity with bleomycin and radiotherapy in oat cell lung cancer. *Cancer* **27**: 2414–2416, 1976.

35. Teilum, G.: Endodermal sinus tumor of the ovary and testis—comparative morphogenesis of the so-called mesonephroma ovarii (Schiller) and extra-embryonic (yolk sac, allantoic) structures of the rat's placenta. *Cancer* **12**:1092–1105, 1959.

36. Teilum, G.: *Special Tumors of Ovary and Testis—Comparative Pathology and Histological Identification.* Copenhagen: Munksgaard and Philadelphia: J. B. Lippincott Co., 1976, p. 33.

37. Talerman, A.: The incidence of yolk sac tumor (endodermal sinus tumor) elements in germ cell tumors of the testis in the adult. *Cancer* **36**:211–215, 1975.

38. Teilmann, I., Kassis, H., and Pietra, G.: Primary germ cell tumor of the anterior mediastinum with features of endodermal sinus tumors. *Acta Pathol Microbiol Scand* **70**: 267–278, 1967.

39. Huntington, R. W., Jr., and Bullock, W. K.: Yolk sac tumors of extragonadal origin. *Cancer* **25**:1357–1367, 1970.

40. Huntington, R. W., Jr., Morgenstern, N. L., Sargent, J. A. Glen, R. N., Richards, A. and Hanford, K. C.: Germinal tumors exhibiting the endodermal sinus pattern of Teilum in young children. *Cancer* **16**:34–47, 1963.

41. Gitlin, D., Pericelli, A., and Gitlin, G. M.: Synthesis of alphafetoprotein by liver, yolk sac, and gastrointestinal tract of the human conceptus. *Cancer Res* **32**:979–982, 1972.

42. Kurman, R. J., and Norris, H. J.: Endodermal sinus tumor of the ovary. *Cancer* **38**: 2404–2419, 1976.

43. Slayton, R. E. Hreshchyshyn, M. M., Silverberg, S. G., Shingleton, H. M., Park, R. C., Disaia, P. J., and Blessing, J. A.: Treatment of malignant ovarian germ cell tumors. *Cancer* **42**:390–398, 1978.

44. Tallerman, A., and Haije, W. G.: Alphafetoprotein and germ cell tumors: a possible role of yolk sac tumor in production of alphafetoprotein. *Cancer* **34**;1722–1726, 1974.

45. Knowles, J. H., and Scully, R. E.: Case records of the Massachusetts General Hospital. Fulminant illness with an abnormal density in the chest. *N Engl J Med* **281**: 434–439, 1969.

INDEX